# Aids to Oral Patholog
# and Diagnosis

CW00558282

CHURCHILL LIVINGSTONE DENTAL BOOKS

# Aids to Oral Pathology and Diagnosis

## R.A. Cawson

MD, FDS RCPS, FRCPath
Professor of Oral Medicine and Pathology,
The United Medical and Dental Schools,
Guy's Hospital, London

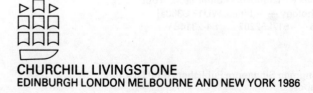

CHURCHILL LIVINGSTONE
EDINBURGH LONDON MELBOURNE AND NEW YORK 1986

CHURCHILL LIVINGSTONE
Medical Division of Longman Group Limited

Distributed in the United States of America by
Churchill Livingstone Inc., 1560 Broadway,
New York, N.Y. 10036, and by associated
companies, branches and representatives
throughout the world.

First published 1981
Second edition 1986

ISBN  0-443-03322-6

**British Library Cataloguing in Publication Data**
Cawson, R.A.
    Aids to oral pathology and diagnosis. —
    2nd ed. — (Aids)
    1. Teeth — Diseases 2. Mouth — Diseases
    I. Title II. Series
    617'.52207 RK307

**Library of Congress Cataloging in Publication Data**
Cawson, R.A.
    Aids to oral pathology and diagnosis.

    (Churchill Livingstone dental books)
    Includes index.
    1. Mouth — Diseases — Outlines, syllabi, etc.
2. Teeth — Diseases — Outlines, syllabi, etc. I. Title.
II. Series. [DNLM: 1. Mouth Diseases — diagnosis —
outlines. 2. Mouth Diseases — pathology — outlines.
3. Tooth Diseases — diagnosis — outlines. 4. Tooth
Diseases — pathology — outlines. WU18 C383a]
RC815.C39 1985     617'.52207     84-23148

Produced by Longman Singapore Publishers (Pte) Ltd.
Printed in Singapore.

# Preface

These Aids are intended to provide summarised information for
revision purposes, for undergraduates and for those sitting the
Fellowship in Dental Surgery. Inevitably, the extent of coverage of
individual topics is uneven but is based on experience of what
students most often seem to find difficult. Nevertheless, some
subjects may have been given too much space.

The scope of these notes goes a little beyond the strict limits of the
title and some aspects of systemic disease which have oral
significance have been included. It also seemed unreasonable not to
include some information about the principles of management of
these conditions — what, after all, is pathology and diagnosis for
except to help treat disease.

Since these notes are for revision purposes any suggestions for
further reading would presumably have come too late.
Bibliographies which might perhaps exacerbate pre-examination
anxiety have therefore been omitted.

I am greatly indebted to Miss Rhona Hickman, Miss Meg Skelly, Dr
John Eveson and Professor Crispian Scully for their helpful
comments, and to Miss Linda van Laere for her patience and skill in
typing and retyping the manuscript.

London, 1986                                          R.A.C.

# Contents

# Contents

# Disorders of development

CAUSES
1. Genetic
2. Acquired

STRUCTURES AFFECTED
1. Teeth
2. Jaws
3. Soft tissues
    (i) Gingivae
    (ii) Mucous membranes
4. Systemic diseases affecting the mouth

## THE TEETH

1. Abnormal numbers
    (i) Simple anodontia or hypodontia
    (ii) Anodontia or hypodontia associated with systemic disorders
    (iii) Additional teeth (hyperdontia)
2. Delayed eruption
    (i) Local obstruction
    (ii) Systemic diseases
3. Defects of structure
    (i) Genetic
    (ii) Acquired
        a. local causes
        b. systemic diseases
4. Morphological anomalies of dental tissues
    Malformed teeth and odontomes

## ABNORMAL NUMBERS OF TEETH

### Simple anodontia and hypodontia
1. Often hereditary (usually autosomal dominant)
2. Third molars, second premolars, maxillary laterals most frequently missing
3. Problems
   (i) If other teeth are lost
   (ii) If there is disparity between sizes of upper and lower arches
   (iii) Cosmetic effects of missing upper laterals

### Anodontia or hypodontia associated with systemic defects

*Ectodermal dysplasia — anhidrotic or hypohidrotic*
1. Genetically determined; mainly males
2. Defects or failure of development of ectodermal structures
3. Hypodontia commoner than anodontia. Teeth usually conical
4. Anodontia. Nutcracker profile, (dentures necessary in childhood)
5. Hair fine and sparse
6. Skin dry (absence of sweat glands). Fingernails often defective

*Down's syndrome (mongolism, trisomy 21)*
1. Hypodontia generally as in normal population but more frequent. Various other teeth often also missing
2. Severe malocclusion — usually class III with anterior open bite
3. Caries usually mild but periodontal disease severe

*Other causes of hypodontia*
1. Cleft palate — teeth in region of defect typically absent or malformed
2. Genetic syndromes of the head and neck. Hypodontia often associated but all rare
3. Pseudohypodontia. Failure of eruption of teeth (as in cleido-cranial dysplasia) or teeth buried by gingival hyperplasia

### Additional teeth — hyperdontia

*Simple hyperdontia*
1. Teeth typically simple conical shape (supernumerary teeth); less often, resemble normal teeth (supplemental teeth)
2. *Supernumerary teeth.* Usually maxillary incisor region. Occasionally midline (mesiodens)
3. *Supplemental teeth.* Supplemental maxillary incisor or premolar least uncommon. Fourth molar rare.

*Syndromes associated with hyperdontia* Main example; cleido-cranial dysplasia. Other disorders even more uncommon

## DELAYED ERUPTION OF TEETH

### Local obstruction to eruption
1. Loss of space
2. Abnormal position of crypt (especially lower third molar and upper canine)
3. Overcrowding
4. Additional teeth
5. Dentigerous cysts
6. Retention of deciduous tooth
7. Eruption cysts. (Probably usually rupture spontaneously)

### Systemic causes (all rare)
1. Metabolic diseases. Cretinism and rickets
2. Osteodystrophies. Cleido-cranial dysplasia and cherubism
3. Hereditary gingival fibromatosis. Apparent failure of eruption — teeth buried by excessive fibrous gingival tissue

### Treatment considerations
1. Radiographs. Ensure that permanent successor is present
2. Make room for tooth by orthodontic means or extractions if necessary
3. Extract buried teeth (mainly mandibular third molars) if infection or other complications develop (see p. 42)

### Complications affecting unerupted or partially erupted teeth
1. Often no clinical effects
2. Pericoronitis (lower 3rd molars)
3. Cyst formation
4. Resorption of adjacent tooth
5. Eruption later under denture
6. Hypercementosis

## DEFECTS OF STRUCTURE OF THE TEETH

### Deciduous teeth
1. Genetic disorders (see below)
2. Acquired disorders
    (i) Fluorosis (only if fluoride content of water excessively high e.g. Northern India)
    (ii) Discolouration by abnormal pigments
        a. Tetracycline (yellow teeth, becoming grey or brown)
        b. Haemolytic jaundice of newborn (yellow or greenish bands of discolouration)
        c. Congenital porphyria (red or purple pigmentation)

**Permanent teeth**

A. Genetic
1. Amelogenesis imperfecta
   (i) Hypoplastic type
   (ii) Hypocalcified type
2. Dentinogenesis imperfecta

B. Acquired
1. Local causes
   Infection of overlying deciduous predecessor
2. Systemic causes
   (i) Infective
      Congenital syphilis
   (ii) Severe disturbances of metabolism
      a. Severe childhood fevers, esp. measles
      b. Rickets and hypoparathyroidism
   (iii) Exogenous causes
      a. Tetracycline
      b. Fluorosis

*Amelogenesis imperfecta*
Characteristically all teeth affected (both dentitions) defects widespread
1. Hereditary enamel hypoplasia
   (i) Various patterns of inheritance
   (ii) Enamel hard and translucent but randomly pitted or very thin
   (iii) Defects become stained but no special susceptibility to caries
2. Hereditary enamel hypocalcification
   (i) Various types of inheritance
   (ii) Enamel weak, opaque and chalky
   (iii) Form normal initially. Soft enamel chips away producing characteristic shouldered form
   (iv) Enamel tends to become yellowish

*Dentinogenesis imperfecta (hereditary opalescent dentine)*
1. Autosomal dominant. Closely related to osteogenesis imperfecta — both may be associated
2. Dentine soft, lacks normal tubular structure
3. Pulp chambers obliterated
4. Roots short; molar crowns bulbous
5. Enamel normal texture, but translucent and brownish or purplish
6. Enamel tends to split off and expose dentine
7. Severe cases — loss of enamel leads to attrition to gum level in early adolescence
8. Crowning impractical, dentures needed in severe cases

*Congenital syphilis*
1. Rare. Defects due to invasion of tooth germ by *Treponema pallidum*
2. Incisors small, tapering with crescentic notch. Often anterior open bite
3. First molars may be dome-shaped (Moon's molars) or have nodular surface (mulberry molars)

*Severe fevers and metabolic disturbances*
Now rare — main examples
1. Measles — Typically horizontal rows of pits or grooves across crown of incisors. Probably due to severe secondary infection
2. Rickets and renal rickets. Hypocalcification — severe cases only
3. Hypoparathyroidism. Ectodermal defects may cause hypoplasia. Defects of nails and absence of hair may be associated

*Tetracycline pigmentation*
1. Tetracycline deposited along incremental lines
2. Teeth initially yellow but become dirty brown or grey. Stain permanent and irremovable
3. Yellow fluorescence under u.v. light (undecalcified section)
4. Appearance disguised by crowning or acid-etch facing

*Note*: No indication for tetracyclines for ordinary childhood infections during period of calcification of teeth, i.e. up to 6th year of childhood

*Fluorosis: mottled enamel*
1. Endemic where waterborne fluoride exceeds 2 ppm
2. Deciduous teeth rarely affected
3. Increased resistance to dental caries, irrespective of severity
4. Grades:
   (i) Very mild — small white opacities of less than 25 per cent of enamel. Normal surface
   (ii) Mild — up to 50 per cent of enamel opaque or stained
   (iii) Moderate — most of enamel patchily opaque white or brown
   (iv) Severe — enamel grossly defective, opaque, pitted, brown and brittle. Skeletal fluorosis (increased radiodensity) may be associated

MORPHOLOGICAL ANOMALIES OF TEETH AND ODONTOMES
Defects range from minor anomalies (e.g. additional cusps) to gross morphological disturbances (odontomes, p. 56)

## DEVELOPMENTAL ANOMALIES OF THE JAWS

Important examples:
1. Micrognathia
2. Macrognathia
3. Cleft lip and palate
4. Cherubism (Familial fibrous dysplasia)
5. Syndrome of multiple jaw cysts and basal cell carcinomas
6. Cleido-cranial dysplasia

## MICROGNATHIA

1. True micrognathia (hypoplasia of jaw or agenesis of condyles) rare
2. False micrognathia — usually post-positioning of normal-size mandible
3. Acquired micrognathia — usually early ankylosis of temporomandibular joint
4. Clinical effects: severe malocclusion and chinless profile

## MACROGNATHIA — PROGNATHISM

1. Hereditary (usually autosomal dominant) or sporadic
2. Relative prognathism (mandibular/maxillary disparity) probably commoner
3. Acquired — acromegaly
4. Clinical consequences — malocclusion and excessively prominent chin. Usually correctable by orthognathic surgery

## CLEFT LIP AND PALATE

1. Causes unknown. Hereditary factors in up to 40 per cent
2. Incidence may exceed 1 : 1000 live births
   Overall male : female ratio about 3 : 2
3. Relative frequencies:
   Cleft lip alone, about 22 per cent
   Cleft lip and palate, about 58 per cent
   Cleft palate alone, about 20 per cent (female : male ratio about 2 : 1)

### Cleft lip (primary palate)

1. Unilateral, with or without alveolar ridge cleft
2. Bilateral, with or without alveolar ridge cleft (either can be complete or incomplete)

### Cleft palate (secondary palate)

1. Bifid uvula
2. Soft palate only
3. Soft and hard palate

**Clefts of lip and palate (Combined defects)**
1. Unilateral (left or right: complete or incomplete)
2. Cleft palate with bilateral cleft lip (complete or incomplete)

*Note*: Lip and anterior alveolar ridge (primary palate) develop before fusion of secondary palate (soft and hard) which fuse from behind forward. Clefts of lip and palate are due to a prolonged disorder of development and more likely to have associated defects of other structures. Clefts of palate can be occult (i.e. lacking bone and/or musculature). Complete clefts extend into nasal cavity

**Associated anomalies**
In about 50 per cent, congenital anomalies (e.g. congenital heart disease, limb defects, spina bifida or mental defects) are associated

**Treatment aspects**
1. Surgical correction usually now possible at about 18 months
2. Speech therapy if necessary
3. Where surgery not feasible, obturator may be used

CHERUBISM (FAMILIAL FIBROUS DYSPLASIA)
1. Usually inherited as simple dominant
2. Typically bilateral soft tissue defects of mandible; sometimes of maxilla. Facial swelling and displacement of teeth in the affected area (p. 66)

SYNDROME OF MULTIPLE JAW CYSTS, BASAL CELL CARCINOMAS AND SKELETAL ANOMALIES
1. Autosomal dominant
2. Mild bossing (especially frontal), broad nasal root, mild hypertelorism, often first signs
3. Basal cell tumours often in childhood or adolescence
4. Radiographs: minor skeletal anomalies e.g. bifid ribs, abnormalities of pituitary fossa, and/or spine, calcification of falx cerebri (in varying combinations)
5. Jaw cysts
   (i) May not appear until adolescence or adulthood
   (ii) Typically keratinise
   (iii) Affect any part of jaws; many (e.g. 5 to 15) may have to be enucleated
6. Warn patient of risks of multiple operations on jaws, of complications of cysts and of treatment of skin tumours

## CLEIDO-CRANIAL DYSPLASIA
1. Rare, autosomal dominant
2. Aplasia or hypoplasia of clavicles, abnormally wide cranium, delayed ossification of fontanelles, excessive numbers of wormian bones
3. Typically small mid-face with depressed nasal bridge; frontal and occipital bossing
4. Prolonged or permanent delay of eruption of many teeth. Many supernumerary teeth (usually remain buried)

## DEVELOPMENTAL ANOMALIES OF ORAL SOFT TISSUES
1. Gingivae. Main example — hereditary fibromatosis
2. Oral mucosa:
    (i) White sponge naevus (p. 79)
    (ii) Epidermolysis bullosa
    (iii) Peutz-Jeghers syndrome
    (iv) Hereditary haemorrhagic telangiectasia
    (v) Ehlers-Danlos syndrome

## EPIDERMOLYSIS BULLOSA
1. Autosomal dominant or recessive
2. Bullae followed by scarring in dystrophic types
3. Dominant dystrophic type. Onset in infancy. Bullae and scarring mainly on extremities and mouth; severity usually decreases with age
4. Simple (recessive) type
    (i) Most common type. Onset in neonatal period
    (ii) Bullae and scarring mainly of face, hands and mouth after minimal trauma
    (iii) Effects — microstomia, tethering and depapillation of tongue, obliteration of sulci
    (iv) Toothbrushing increases blistering — periodontal disease and/or caries often rampant
    (v) Enamel may be hypoplastic
    (vi) Sometimes blisters of other mucous membranes (e.g. eyes or larynx) with scarring
5. Some response to phenytoin — may help to allow dentistry to be done

## PEUTZ-JEGHERS SYNDROME
1. Autosomal dominant
2. Melanotic macules (freckles) peri-and intra-orally, and on face
3. Skin pigment fades gradually; may be absent in adults
4. Associated hamartomatous polyps of gastrointestinal tract — mainly small intestine. Not premalignant but can cause intussusception or obstruction

## HEREDITARY HAEMORRHAGIC TELANGIECTASIA
1. Autosomal dominant but onset usually in adult life
2. Pinhead or spider-like telangiectases of mouth, face, head and sometimes of viscera
3. Severe epistaxis often early
4. Sometimes oral bleeding especially from lips or tongue
5. Haemostatic function normal. No special risks with extractions

## EHLERS-DANLOS SYNDROME
1. Nine subtypes (some inherited as autosomal dominants) with different collagen defects
2. Typical features
   (i) Hyperelastic skin
   (ii) Fragility of mucosa and skin with easy bruising and gaping of wounds
   (iii) Often hypermobility of joints
   (iv) Teeth — roots deformed, multiple pulp stones
   (v) Early-onset periodontitis (periodontosis) in Type VIII

## GENETIC SYSTEMIC DISORDERS AFFECTING DENTAL PATIENTS

1. Cyclic neutropenia (p. 111)
2. Haemophilia (p. 108)
3. Von Willebrand's disease (p. 109)
4. Malignant hyperpyrexia

# Dental caries

## AETIOLOGY

1. Cariogenic bacteria
2. Frequent supply of substrate (sugar)
3. Host factors including susceptible tooth surfaces

## MICROBIOLOGICAL ASPECTS

### 1. Evidence of infective nature of caries:
   (i) Caries fails to develop in germ-free animals on potentially cariogenic (high sugar) diets
   (ii) Caries develops when cariogenic bacteria are inoculated into mouths of germ-free animals (making them gnotobiotes) given high sugar diet
   (iii) Caries significantly reduced in humans and animals taking long-term antibiotics

### 2. Important properties of cariogenic bacteria:
   (i) Adhere to enamel surface
   (ii) Form insoluble polysaccharides (glucans) as plaque matrix from sucrose especially
   (iii) Form acid from dietary substrate (sugar)
   (iv) Survive and continue metabolism at low pH

### 3. *Streptococcus mutans* strains
   (i) Some highly cariogenic for animals
   (ii) Preferential adherence to hard surfaces
   (iii) Colonization of tooth surface favoured by high sucrose diet
   (iv) Cariogenic strains produce insoluble polysaccharides (glucans or mutans) from sucrose by action of glucosyl transferases
   (v) Able to maintain acid production at lower pH and lower optimal pH for growth than most streptococci

(vi) Epidemiological association of *Strep. mutans* with human caries, not consistent finding

(vii) High sucrose diets frequently associated with increased population of *Strep. mutans* and increased caries in humans and animals

## 4. Other streptococci

(i) *Streptococcus sanguis.* More effective than *Strep. mutans* at colonising tooth surfaces. Some strains cariogenic for animals and possibly humans

(ii) *Strep. mitior* produces mainly intra-cellular (storage) polysaccharides. Some strains cariogenic for animals

(iii) *Strep. salivarius.* Preferential affinity for soft tissues. Usually forms soluble (levan-like) polysaccharides. Probably not cariogenic

(iv) *Strep. milleri.* Highly cariogenic in animals

## 5. Lactobacilli

(i) Many species. Fastidious growth requirements. Types of acids produced also vary. *L. acidophilus* isolated from carious cavity at pH 3.5

(ii) More lactobacilli in saliva than plaque

(iii) Some strains produce glucans; proliferation favoured by high sugar diet

(iv) Some lactobacilli cariogenic for animals (mainly fissure lesions)

(v) Lactobacilli probably often secondary invaders

(vi) Some association with caries in man (genus not intensively investigated)

(vii) Lactobacillus count of saliva — no predictive value for caries activity

## 6. Actinomyces (*A. viscosus* and *A. naeslundii*)

(i) Present in plaque in large numbers

(ii) Many properties necessary for cariogenesis but may produce less fall in pH

(iii) Cause caries, particularly of root surfaces, in animals and possibly man

## Comments

1. Precise microbial cause of caries in man cannot be established with certainty

2. Circumstantial evidence suggests that strains of *Strep. mutans* are probably the main cariogenic bacteria in man

3. Several types of bacteria, alone or in combination, may be able to cause caries in man under favourable circumstances

BACTERIAL PLAQUE
 1. Primary, non-bacterial pellicle formed by deposition of salivary glycoproteins in presence of calcium
 2. Streptococci typically *Strep. sanguis* colonise pellicle early
 3. Filamentous bacteria (the most prominent histological feature of plaque) follow after about 5 to 7 days, but role unknown
 4. Plaque flora ultimately complex and respiration predominantly anaerobic
 5. Extra-cellular materials, particularly polysaccharides, form about 30 per cent of plaque
 6. Plaque polysaccharides
    (i) Mediate bacterial adhesion
    (ii) Form matrix of plaque
    (iii) May act as a diffusion barrier against escape of acids or entry of buffers
    (iv) Provide bacterial nutrient reserves
 7. Acid production in plaque (Stephan curve)
    (i) Brief exposure to sugar causes rapid fall in pH
    (ii) After 5–10 minutes, pH may be low enough to decalcify enamel
    (iii) pH can remain at critical level for about 20 minutes
    (iv) Slow return to resting level after about 45 minutes
 8. pH levels in plaque mainly depend on:
    (i) Frequency of availability of sugar to bacteria
    (ii) Rate of diffusion of sugar into plaque
    (iii) Rate of sugar metabolism in plaque
    (iv) Rate of diffusion of acid out of plaque
    (v) Buffer production in plaque
    (vi) Buffer production by saliva
    (vii) Diffusion of salivary buffers into plaque
 9. Effect of thickness of plaque
    (i) Clinically, caries develops only where plaque forms thickly (stagnation areas)
    (ii) Undisturbed plaque in stagnation areas may have more cariogenic bacterial population
    (iii) Thick plaque impedes salivary buffering and escape of acids from tooth surfaces
10. Other (possibly protective) components of plaque
    (i) Fluoride (concentrated in plaque)
    (ii) Phosphates
    (iii) Calcium salts
    (iv) Immunoglobulins

11. Evidence of importance of plaque in caries production
    (i) Strains of *Strep. mutans* producing insoluble glucans
        (mutans) are cariogenic in animals
    (ii) Caries develops only where plaque forms thickly (stagnation
        areas)
    (iii) Cervical caries can be stopped by removal of plaque
    (iv) Experimentally, caries prevented in animals by enzymes
        (dextranases) inhibiting glucan production

## BACTERIAL SUBSTRATE

### Role of sugar (sucrose)

*1. Animal experiments*
    (i) High sugar diet essential for high caries activity
    (ii) Sucrose cariogenic locally in mouth, but not when given by
        gastric tube

*2. Epidemiological evidence in humans*
    (i) Low caries activity associated with low sugar ('primitive') diets
    (ii) Rapid increase in caries prevalence with rapid increase in
        sugar intake (mid 19th century) in UK
    (iii) Low caries activity associated with sugar shortages in World
        War II
    (iv) In hereditary fructose intolerance, sugar intake and caries
        activity at very low levels

*3. Clinical evidence*
    (i) Vipeholm caries study — high caries activity only with high
        (adhesive) sugar content
    (ii) Turku xylitol study — caries reduced by about 90 per cent
        when xylitol substituted for sugar
    *Note*: In all above circumstances, low caries activity (on low sugar
    diets) *in spite of normal or high intake of starches*

*4. Microbiological importance of sucrose*
    (i) High sugar intake favours colonisation and proliferation of
        *Strep. mutans*
    (ii) Acid rapidly produced from sugars by *Strep. mutans* and
        other bacteria
    (iii) Rapid and prolonged fall in pH of plaque in *situ* when exposed
        to sugar
    (iv) Sucrose polymerised directly to form insoluble glucans
        essential for matrix of cariogenic plaque

5. *Quantitative and qualitative aspects of sugar and caries*
   (i) Decalcification of tooth depends on persistently low pH
  (ii) Persistently low pH achieved by
     a. Frequent intake of sugar (sweets, etc.)
     b. adhesiveness of sweet foods (e.g. caramels) causing
       prolonged release of sugar to plaque
  (iii) Importance of frequency of intake and adhesiveness (slow
     clearance) of sugars confirmed by
     a. animal experiments
     b. Vipeholm study in humans
  (iv) Overall *quantity* of sugar eaten determines *frequency* with
     which it can be eaten
   (v) In practical terms, sucrose is most important cariogenic
     substrate but glucose and fructose also cariogenic

6. *Starches*
   (i) Relatively inaccessible to plaque bacteria
   (ii) Very low cariogenicity in themselves but
  (iii) Can increase cariogenicity when combined with sugar, by
     making mixture more adhesive
  (iv) No evidence of protective effect of whole wheat products (e.g.
     wholemeal bread)

## HOST FACTORS
1. Salivary activities
2. Immune responses
3. Susceptibility of tooth surface

## SALIVA
1. Caries activity much increased in xerostomia; affects areas of
   teeth not otherwise susceptible
2. Xerostomia
   (i) Delays clearance of foodstuffs from teeth
   (ii) Favours proliferation of *Strep. mutans*
  (iii) Reduces buffering power of saliva
  (iv) Reduces salivary immunoglobulins reaching mouth
3. Rate of flow and buffering power
   (i) High flow rates and bicarbonate buffering interrelated
   (ii) High flow rates and buffering power tend to be associated
     with lower caries activity, e.g. Down's syndrome
4. Saliva and plaque formation
   (i) Primary (non-bacterial) pellicle formed by deposition of
     glycoproteins
   (ii) Salivary proteins in plaque may assist interbacterial
     adhesion
5. Factors with *possible* protective functions
   (i) Lysozyme
   (ii) Thiocyanate and lactoperoxidase
  (iii) Immunoglobulins and complement

## IMMUNE RESPONSES
1. IgA in saliva (main oral antibody). Traces of IgG and IgM from gingival exudate
2. Antibodies against *Strep. mutans* (and other oral bacteria) detectable in serum, saliva and gingival exudate
3. Findings relating antibody levels to caries activity conflicting
4. No firm evidence that natural immunity (high antibody titres) will prevent cariogenic diet from causing caries in humans
5. Findings relating to caries activity in immunodeficiency disorders (especially IgA deficiency), conflicting but low caries activity in Down's syndrome despite multiple immunodeficiencies
6. Immunisation of animals with anti-*Strep. mutans* vaccines frequently (but not invariably) effective against *Strep. mutans* caries
7. Mechanism of protection and variable responses to immunisation of animals not fully understood
8. Possibility of immunisation of humans against caries dependent on:
    (i) Establishing precise microbial cause of caries in humans
    (ii) Effectiveness of vaccine in preventing activity of *all* bacteria capable of causing caries
    (iii) *Absolute certainty* that vaccine has no side-effects worse than the disease, either systemic or local


## SUSCEPTIBILITY OF TOOTH SURFACE
1. Susceptibility of tooth surface not distinguishable from oral environmental factors *in vivo*
2. Post-eruptive changes
    (i) Teeth most susceptible immediately after eruption
    (ii) Newly erupted teeth can absorb 10 to 20 times as much inorganic material as mature teeth
    (iii) Absorption of (unknown) factors after eruption may be protective
3. Developmental and nutritional aspects
    (i) No evidence that hypocalcification (vitamin D deficiency or hereditary) increases caries susceptibility
    (ii) No evidence that any other deficiency or developmental defects (e.g. enamel hypoplasia) increase caries susceptibility
4. *Only fluorides known for certain to be protective*
5. Mechanism of fluoride protection controversial. May be by:
    (i) Incorporation into forming enamel
    (ii) More stable crystalline lattice of fluorapatite may increase resistance to dissolution by acid
    (iii) Fluoride in plaque may promote remineralisation when caries initiated
    (iv) High concentrations of fluoride may affect plaque metabolism

6. Genetic aspects
   (i) Animals can be bred for caries susceptibility
   (ii) Nature of this genetic susceptibility unknown
   (iii) Little evidence of *significant* genetic effect on caries
         susceptibility in humans

## PATHOLOGY OF DENTAL CARIES

ENAMEL CARIES
Microscopic and sub-microscopic phases
   (i) Initiation (sub-microscopic damage)
   (ii) Bacterial invasion
   (iii) Secondary enamel caries
1. Initiation phase. Conical, multi-zone lesion, with apex deeply
   (i) Peripheral translucent zone
   (ii) Dark zone
   (iii) Body of lesion
   (iv) Surface zone
2. Surface zone; more radiopaque and enhanced striae of Retzius
3. Deeper zones due to demineralisation and formation of sub-
   microscopic pores resulting from permeation of enamel by acid
   from plaque. Polarised light studies allow pore sizes to be
   assessed by means of their ability to imbibe media with molecules
   of known size. Amount of decalcification in each zone assessed by
   microradiography
4. Protein matrix keratin-like
5. Hydrogen ions permeate matrix to reach surfaces of enamel
   crystals. No evidence of preferential dissolution of protein matrix
6. Tissue destruction eventually allows bacterial invasion
7. Secondary enamel caries
   (i) Lateral spread of bacteria along amelodentinal junction
   (ii) Enamel attacked from beneath and undermined
   (iii) Widespread disintegration

CARIES OF DENTINE
1. Initial changes non-bacterial but due to diffusion of acid via
   porous enamel
2. Acid spreads laterally along amelodentinal junction and deeply
   via tubules, producing conical lesion
3. Later, pioneer bacteria (gram-positive cocci) spread down tubules
4. Tubules eventually filled and distended with bacteria
5. Dissolution of intervening decalcified dentine forms liquefaction
   foci. Progressive destruction follows

REACTIONS OF DENTINE AND PULP
1. Pulpal reaction initiated by penetration of acid before bacterial
   invasion

2. Dead tracts. Odontoblasts killed. Empty tubules dark to transmitted light. Calcified tissue seals off affected tubules
3. Translucent zones. At margins of dead tracts or under very slow caries or attrition. Continued calcification (peritubular dentine) until tubule obliterated. Dentine becomes homogeneous and impermeable
4. Regular secondary dentine forms under slowly progressive caries, attrition or abrasion
5. Irregular secondary dentine forms under more acute lesions — tubules few, irregular or absent
6. Pulpitis — initially 'sterile', i.e. due to acid; later infected

**Diagnostic aspects**
1. Sites of attack
   (i) Occlusal pits and fissures
   (ii) Interstitially
   (iii) Cervical margins
2. Early occlusal caries. Softening of walls of fissures causes probe to stick
3. Early interstitial caries. Detectable radiographically
4. Acute caries. Typically children. Small visible cavity, widely undermined enamel and dentine rapidly penetrated; little secondary dentine. Early exposure
5. Chronic caries. Typically adults. Slow penetration. Extensive secondary dentine. Exposure late

# Pulpitis, periapical periodontitis and injuries to the teeth

## PULPITIS

### Causes
1. Dental caries
2. Traumatic exposure
3. Fracture of crown
4. Thermal injury
5. Chemical injury
6. Cracked tooth syndrome

### Histological types of pulpitis
1. Closed pulpitis ranges from hyperaemia to abscess formation or cellulitis. Inflammatory infiltrate dependent on acuteness of the process
   (i) Acute — usually diffuse, leading to necrosis
   (ii) Chronic — typically localised, sometimes with abscess formation
2. Open pulpitis — chronic inflammation and proliferation

### Symptoms
1. Acute pulpitis
   (i) Early hypersensitivity to hot or cold
   (ii) Severe spontaneous lancinating pain
   (iii) Death of pulp may be followed by acute apical periodontitis
2. Chronic pulpitis
   (i) Hypersensitivity to extremes of hot or cold
   (ii) Spontaneous pain absent or fugitive, *poorly localised*, intermittent over long period

   *Note*: Symptoms not reliably related to microscopic changes

### Diagnosis
1. Look for deep caries particularly under restorations
2. Look for deep restorations, possibly involving pulp, on radiographs
3. Test suspected teeth with electric tester and with heat and cold
4. Remove doubtful restorations if necessary

18

**Possible managements**
1. Preservation of vital pulp (capping or pulpotomy)
2. Pulpectomy and root canal treatment
3. Extraction

## CRACKED TOOTH SYNDROME
1. Hairline crack in apparently sound tooth (especially premolar) or beside restoration
2. Exposure of pulp via crack — acute pulpitis or symptomless pulp death and acute periodontitis
3. Pressure with ball burnisher to force apart cusps, transillumination or use of dye may demonstrate crack

## OPEN PULPITIS
1. Gross exposure but survival of pulp
2. Proliferation of granulation tissue
3. Epithelialisation and fibrosis
4. Symptomless but may be visible as pulp polyp

**Restorative procedures**

*Causes of physical and chemical injuries to the pulp*:
1. Thermal injury (e.g. overheating during cavity preparation, large unlined metal restorations)
2. Chemical injury: irritant restorative materials (cements containing phosphoric acid, self-curing resins with free monomer)
   Pulp damage often , however, due to poor peripheral seal and permeation by bacteria
3. Mechanical injury (exposure)

*Histological effects (according to severity of injury)*:
1. Disorganisation of odontoblast layer
2. Oedema ('blistering') of odontoblast layer
3. Death of odontoblasts
4. Secondary dentine
5. Pulpitis
6. Death of pulp

## DEGENERATIVE CHANGES IN THE PULP
1. Fatty change
2. Fibrosis
3. Diffuse calcification
   Probably due to progressive ischaemia but not clinically detectable or significant

## PULP STONES
1. Developmental anomaly
2. No clinical significance except when obstructing root canal treatment

## PERIAPICAL PERIODONTITIS

### Causes
1. Infection (usually from caries and pulpitis)
2. Trauma (usually with death of pulp)
3. Chemical injury

### Pathology
1. Source of infection
   (i) Root canal (most cases)
   (ii) Periodontal pocket (probable source in absence of caries)
2. Usually low grade chronic infection localised by periapical inflammatory and immune response
3. Possible routes of spread of infection (if more virulent)
   (i) Gingival discharge (sinus)
   (ii) Skin discharge (sinus)
   (iii) Spread along medulla (osteomyelitis)
   (iv) Spread into adjacent fascial spaces and beyond (cellulitis)
4. Epithelial content
   (i) Rests of Malassez proliferate (unless destroyed by infection)
   (ii) Periapical cyst may form
5. Healing of chronic lesions
   (i) Depends on debridement and obliteration of root canal or removal of tooth
   (ii) No spontaneous healing otherwise

### ACUTE APICAL PERIODONTITIS
1. Microbiology — no specific pathogens
2. Typical acute inflammatory reaction
   (i) Neutrophil exudate
   (ii) Pus formation
   (iii) Osteoclastic resorption of periapical bone
   (iv) Resorption of cortical bone (sometimes)
   (v) Rarely, spread within bone (osteomyelitis)

### Diagnosis
   (i) Severe, well-localised, throbbing pain
   (ii) Tenderness of tooth in socket
   (iii) No response to vitality tests
   (iv) Minimal widening of periapical space on radiographs (unless acute-on-chronic)
   (v) Oedema of face if infection spreads through cortex
   (vi) Regional lymphadenopathy

### Management
   (i) Open and drain root canal. Fill when quiescent, OR
   (ii) Extract
   (iii) No justification for antibiotics in healthy patients unless drainage or extraction has to be delayed

CHRONIC PERIODONTITIS (PERIAPICAL GRANULOMA)
1. Microbiology — no specific pathogens
2. Typical chronic inflammatory reaction
   (i) Mononuclear cells predominant
  (ii) Proliferation of granulation tissue
 (iii) Resorption of surrounding bone
 (iv) Variable central epithelial proliferation
  (v) Suppuration — chronic gingival or skin sinus
 (vi) Periodontal cyst formation in some cases
(vii) Local immune response helps to localise the lesion

### Diagnosis
  (i) Often no symptoms
 (ii) Tooth may be slightly tender
(iii) No response to vitality tests
(iv) Round periapical radiolucency

### Management
  (i) Root fill (granulomas or small cysts heal spontaneously) OR
 (ii) Extract
(iii) Periapical surgery only for failed endodontic treatment

*Note*: Root canal treatment justified only if crown is restorable and the rest of dentition healthy

## INJURIES TO TEETH AND SUPPORTING TISSUES

1. Fractures of crown
2. Fractures of root
3. Injuries to pulp
  (i) In fracture of crown
 (ii) Tearing of apical vessels (without fracture)
4. Injury to periodontal membrane
  (i) Temporary periodontitis
 (ii) Irreversible destruction of attachment
5. Injuries to supporting bone
  (i) Fracture of socket edge
 (ii) Fracture of alveolar ridge
6. Injuries to adjacent soft tissues
7. Injury to developing teeth — dilaceration
8. Chronic injuries to teeth
  (i) Attrition
 (ii) Abrasion
(iii) Erosion

## ACUTE INJURIES

**General aspects of diagnosis**
1. Other injuries, especially to skull or to perioral tissues?
2. Emotional state? — delay treatment if shocked or sedate if necessary
3. Dental aspects
    (i) History
       a. Nature of and time since accident
       b. Pain — pulpal or periodontal?
    (ii) Clinical examination
       a. General state of dentition?
       b. Conserve teeth if possible and if state of dentition justifies
       c. Test response of pulps
       d. Extent of fracture. Look for exposure or longitudinal splits
       e. Periodontal state. Mobility (without fracture) — root or bone fractures, or major periodontal membrane tear — apical vessels often severed
    (iii) Radiographs for
       a. Stage of root development
       b. Any root fracture and its position
       c. Widening of periodontal membrane space
       d. Fracture of alveolar process
       e. Damage to other teeth
       f. Any coincidental pathology
       g. Late cases — apical periodontitis

**Principles of management**

*Class I:*   Traumatised tooth without fracture
      1. No displacement
         Apical vessels often torn, death of pulp frequently
         asymptomatic. Effects often long delayed
      2. Loosened teeth. Manipulate into position. Splint

*Class II:*   Fracture of crown
      1. Enamel only. Repair defect. Test vitality at intervals
      2. Enamel and dentine. Protect open tubules with Ca(OH)$_2$
         and temporary crown
         Splint any loosening or displacement

*Class III:*   Coronal fracture with exposure (or near exposure) of pulp
      1. Exposure with open apex
         No apparent infection — pulp cap or vital pulpotomy
         Non-vital pulp — pulpectomy, apical dressing with
         CaOH$_2$, root fill later
      2. Exposure with closed apex
         Root fill

*Class IV:*   Fracture of root
      1. Coronal third
         Extract
      2. Apical third
         Splint (may heal by cemental scar); test vitality at
         intervals

*Class V:*   Avulsion of tooth
      1. Space maintenance — replace later *or*
      2. Replant if recent case
         Wash, replace and splint. Root fill later only if necessary

RESORPTION AND HYPERCEMENTOSIS

(*Note*: Apical periodontitis is most common cause of minor
resorption and/or cementosis but rarely clinically significant)

**Resorption**

*Complications of physiological resorption of deciduous teeth*
1. Ankylosis
2. Separation of apex
3. Failure of resorption (successor usually absent)

*Causes of resorption of permanent teeth*
1. Apical periodontitis
2. Pressure of adjacent impacted tooth
3. Neoplasms
4. Unerupted teeth (late change)
5. Replanted teeth
6. Idiopathic
   (i) Generalised (external) resorption — usually apical
   (ii) Internal (pink spot — sometimes history of trauma)

## Pathology

1. Typical giant cell (osteoclastic) hard tissue destruction
2. Variable associated reparative changes

## Hypercementosis

*Causes*

1. Apical periodontitis (usually with resorption nearby)
2. Ageing
3. Unerupted teeth (often with some resorption)
4. Paget's disease of jaws (p. 65)
5. Cementomas (p. 57)
   Usually no clinical significance but, if gross, can interfere with extraction

# Periodontal disease (gingivitis and periodontitis)

GINGIVITIS
1. Acute ulcerative gingivitis (acute necrotising ulcerative gingivitis, ANUG, Vincent's gingivitis)
2. Acute herpetic gingivostomatitis
3. Chronic marginal gingivitis

PERIODONTITIS
1. Acute periodontitis
2. Chronic periodontitis (horizontal or vertical bone loss types)
3. Juvenile periodontitis (periodontosis)

OTHER GINGIVAL DISORDERS
1. Gingival hyperplasia
   (i) Hereditary
   (ii) Phenytoin-induced
2. Recession (atrophy)
   (i) Localised
   (ii) Generalised

## ACUTE ULCERATIVE GINGIVITIS

**Microbiology**
1. Anaerobic infection (responds to metronidazole)
2. Overwhelming proliferation of *Fusobacterium nucleatum* and *Borrelia vincentii*

**Associated factors**
1. Poor oral hygiene
2. Smoking
3. 'Stress'
4. Upper respiratory infections

**Pathology**
Invasion of tissues by spirochetes. Acute inflammation, destruction of gingival epithelium and connective tissue

**Clinical features**
1. Otherwise healthy young adults (not children)
2. Spontaneous gingival bleeding and soreness. Systemic upset or lymphadenitis uncommon
3.    a. cratered ulcers of interdental papillae with yellowish-grey slough and plaque accumulation
     b. spread along gingival margins. Deep extension destroys interdental tissues if untreated
4. Contact ulceration of mucosa rare
5. Little or no systemic effects. Rarely, lymphadenopathy
6. Management — rapid response to thorough debridement of plaque and metronidazole (200 mg thrice daily for three days)
7. May recur. Follow-up to maintain better oral hygiene

**Diagnosis**
1. Clinical features (see above)
2. Smear shows little else but Fusobacteria, spirochaetes and leucocytes

## ACUTE HERPETIC GINGIVOSTOMATITIS

1. Redness and oedema of gingivae. Sometimes ulcerated
2. Randomly distributed vesicles and ulcers, sometimes also on gingivae (p. 71)
3. Lymphadenopathy and systemic upset often severe
4. Children decreasingly affected

## CHRONIC MARGINAL GINGIVITIS

See page 27

## ACUTE PERIODONTITIS

**Causes**
1. Traumatic. Blow on tooth. Contusion or tearing of periodontal fibres. Temporary pain and tenderness
2. Periodontal (lateral) abscess (see below)
3. Ulcerative gingivitis. In severe or untreated cases, destruction of interdental gingiva, alveolar bone, periodontal membrane (see above)

## CHRONIC GINGIVITIS AND PERIODONTITIS

### Aetiology
1. Gingivitis caused by accumulation of plaque; abolished by removal of plaque
2. Destruction of supporting tissues (periodontitis) typically follows long-standing gingivitis but relationship variable and complicated by other factors
3. Progress depends on balance between virulence of plaque bacteria and host responses

### Microbiology of plaque
1. Role of individual pathogens of plaque difficult to evaluate
2. Human plaque bacteria able to cause periodontal destruction in animals include:
    - (i) *Actinomyces viscosus* and *A. naeslundii* (some strains)
    - (ii) *Bacteroides asaccharolyticus (gingivalis)*
    - (iii) *Capnocytophaga (Bacteroides ochraceus)*
    - (iv) *Eikenella corrodens*
    - (v) *Fusobacterium nucleatum*
    - (vi) *Selenomonas sputigena*
    - (vii) *Strep. mutans* (some strains)
    - (viii) *Actinobacillus actinomycetemcomitans*
3. In humans severe destruction tends to be associated with increased numbers of gram-negative anaerobes
4. Calculus. Deposition of calcium salts from saliva or gingival exudate in plaque and calcifying bacteria (e.g. *Bacterionema matruchottii*)

### Animal experiments
1. Bacterial plaque in animals often not associated with periodontal disease
2. Implantation of many human plaque bacteria (see above) into germ-free animals induces severe periodontal destruction
3. Gram-positive bacteria. Typically cause heavy plaque formation and bone destruction but few osteoclasts
4. Gram-negative bacteria cause bone destruction, many osteoclasts, minimal plaque
5. No significant inflammatory reaction or lymphocytic infiltrates in periodontal tissues in these infections
6. Periodontal destruction apparently directly due to bacteria. Some (e.g. strains of *A. viscosus*) produce bone-resorbing factors

**Host responses — immunological aspects**
1. Many plaque bacteria or their products are antigenic — antibodies or cell-mediated immunity produced as *natural response*
2. Immune reactions to plaque bacteria may be protective but, *hypothetically*, may mediate tissue damage
3. Complexes of antigen and antibody or aggregated immune globulins or endotoxin can activate complement to produce mediators of inflammation
4. *Postulated* mechanisms of immunologically mediated periodontal injury
    (i) Immediate hypersensitivity — IgE mediated release of mediators from mast cells
   (ii) Cytotoxic injury
  (iii) Immune complex injuries
  (iv) Cell-mediated. Release of lymphokines (e.g. osteoclast activating factor), lymphocytotoxins or macrophage collagenase

**Immunological aspects of human periodontal disease**
1. Lymphocyte activation (transformation), antibody production (B cells) or cell-mediated immunity (T cells) are *normal* responses to plaque antigens
2. Complement activation may contribute to gingivitis (but no evidence that inflammation *causes* periodontal destruction)
3. Periodontal destruction not dependent on inflammation, e.g. periodontosis and gnotobiotic infections (see above)
4. Immunosuppressive drugs suppress clinical signs of *gingivitis* (by anti-inflammatory action) but no evidence that destructive changes are reduced
5. In natural immunodeficiency states periodontal destruction can be early and rapid (e.g. Down's syndrome)
6. Conflicting reports of levels of cell-mediated immunity and severity of human periodontal disease
7. Delayed 'hypersensitivity' is a clinical indicator of cell-mediated immunity — not *per se* an indicator of cell-mediated tissue injury and frequently associated with increased *resistance* to infection (e.g. tuberculosis)
8. Human plaque pathogens produce severe periodontal destruction in animals but *no* significant immunocyte response and cell-mediated immunity may be diminished
9. Currently no direct or clinical evidence that periodontal destruction is immunologically mediated in humans
10. Immunological findings have no implications for treatment

## Pathology
1. Plaque on tooth surface
2. Predominantly mononuclear inflammatory infiltrate (lymphocytes and plasma cells) localised to vicinity of plaque
3. Inflammatory gingival swelling (variable false pocket formation)
4. Destruction of periodontal ligament
5. Resorption of alveolar bone
6. Rootward migration of epithelial attachment
7. True pockets formed by destruction of supporting tissues but preservation of gingival connective tissue and epithelium
8. Bone resorption may be uniform around the arch (horizontal bone loss). Severe (vertical) bone loss around individual teeth due to complicating factors (often unidentifiable)
9. Intra-bony pockets formed by destruction of attachment to levels apical to crest of bone
10. Progressive destruction of attachment leads to loosening of teeth

## Diagnosis
1. Plaque. Increased accumulation due to:
   (i) Poor oral hygiene
   (ii) Irregularities of teeth
   (iii) Partial dentures, bridges or faulty restorations
2. Gingivitis. Redness, bleeding and oedema
3. Periodontitis
   (i) Gingivitis
   (ii) True pocketing
   (iii) Bone loss on radiographs (vertical or horizontal)
   (iv) Subgingival calculus
   (v) Alteration of gingival contour
   (vi) Increasing mobility of teeth

## General principles of management
1. Debridement of plaque and calculus
2. Establish effective oral hygiene habits
3. When loss of attachment and pocketing develop surgical treatment may be justified
   Root planing probably most effective and least disfiguring

## PREGNANCY GINGIVITIS
1. Exacerbation of pre-existing gingivitis
2. Sometimes localised proliferation of oedematous vascular connective tissue (pregnancy epulis)
3. Regression post-partum with adequate oral hygiene. If not — excise

## PERIODONTAL (LATERAL) ABSCESS
1. Usually a complication of advanced periodontal disease
2. Possibly due to injury to pocket floor (e.g. food packing) or more virulent infection
3. Acute inflammation deeply in pocket; heavy neutrophil infiltration, rapid osteoclastic resorption of bony floor and wall
4. Pain and tenderness of tooth and gum. Pus may point on attached gingiva or at gingival margin. Deep pocket. Tooth vital
5. Management — drainage. Elective surgery

## GINGIVAL SWELLING

### Fibrous hyperplasia
1. Hereditary
2. Drug-associated
    a. Phenytoin
    b. Cyclosporin

### Inflammatory
1. Chronic oedematous ('hyperplastic') gingivitis
2. Pregnancy gingivitis
3. Leukaemic gingivitis (p. 110)
4. Wegener's granulomatosis (p. 122)
5. Severe scurvy

## GINGIVAL RECESSION

### Localised
1. Anatomical (inadequate tissue overlying root)
2. High frenal attachment

### Generalised
1. Wear and tear ('senile') e.g. over-vigorous toothbrushing
2. Destructive
    (i) Severe ulcerative gingivitis
    (ii) Advanced chronic periodontitis (some cases)
    (iii) Eosinophilic granuloma — rare but may be presenting feature (p. 61)

## GINGIVAL HYPERPLASIA

### Hereditary
1. Autosomal dominant
2. Generalised smooth fibrous thickening of gingivae. May bury teeth
3. Deep false pockets but typically no inflammation
4. Associated features — hirsutism, thickened facial features sometimes. Mental retardation and epilepsy occasionally
5. Management — gingivectomy delayed, preferably until after puberty

### Drug-associated
1. Proliferation of subgingival collagen mainly of interdental papillae
2. Interdental papillae grossly swollen, pale, firm, enhanced orange-peel stippling. Often not inflamed
3. Improve plaque control
4. Gingivectomy if required; repeated as necessary

## PERIODONTOSIS (JUVENILE PERIODONTITIS)

1. Rapid loss of periodontal attachment starting in childhood or teens
2. Initial non-inflammatory stage controversial but periodontosis occasionally due to systemic defect where periodontal membrane structure may be defective, e.g. Ehlers-Danlos syndrome
3. Suggested aetiology
   (i) Specific plaque pathogens, e.g. *Capnocytophaga* and/or
   (ii) Neutrophil defect, or
   (iii) Defect of cell-mediated immunity
4. Typically, permanent teeth affected, especially incisors and 1st molars
5. Severe pocketing and vertical bone destruction. Teeth may be lost in teens or 20s
6. Earlier stages may respond to vigorous treatment

## OTHER CAUSES OR EARLY-ONSET PERIODONTAL DESTRUCTION

1. Immunodeficiency disorders
   a. Down's syndrome
   b. Uncontrolled diabetes mellitus
   c. Leucopenia (any cause)
2. Genetic syndromes
   a. Hypophosphatasia
   b. Hyperkeratosis palmaris et plantaris
   c. Ehlers Danlos syndrome type VIII
3. Eosinophilic granuloma (histiocytosis X)

## HYPERKERATOSIS PALMARIS ET PLANTARIS WITH PERIODONTOSIS (PAPILLON LEFEVRE SYNDROME)

1. Autosomal recessive
2. Keratosis (scaling) of palms and feet precede oral changes
3.  (i) Gingivae become red and swollen soon after eruption of teeth
    (ii) Progressive destruction of periodontal ligament and pocket
         formation (both dentitions)
    (iii) All teeth usually lost in teens. No residual defects in mouth
    (iv) Pathogenesis of periodontal damage unknown

## CAUSES OF MAJOR GINGIVAL OR PERIODONTAL SYMPTOMS

GINGIVAL BLEEDING

**Local**
1. Chronic gingivitis
2. Acute ulcerative gingivitis

**Systemic**

*Purpura* (p. 107)
1. Acute leukaemia
2. Idiopathic thrombocytopenic
3. Scurvy
4. Drug-induced

LOOSENING OF THE TEETH

1. Chronic periodontal disease
2. Periodontosis
3. Periodontal (lateral) abscess
4. Fracture of root
5. Fracture of alveolar bone
6. Acute osteomyelitis
7. Malignant tumours of jaw
8. Histiocytosis X

# Epidemiological aspects of oral disease

## SOME OBJECTIVES OF EPIDEMIOLOGICAL STUDIES
1. To determine incidence or prevalence of disease
2. To seek factors affecting prevalence or distribution of disease as a guide to aetiology
3. To seek preventive measures applicable to the community
4. To assess need and demand for care
5. To evaluate community treatment or preventive measures

*Note*: *Incidence* is the number of *new* cases of a disease, per unit of population (e.g. per 100 000), in a given period, i.e. the 'attack rate'

*Prevalence* of disease is the proportion of the population affected by the disease at a given time and is a product of both incidence and duration of the disease. The prevalence of dental caries or periodontal disease is thus considerably easier to measure than the incidence.

## SOME SOURCES OF DATA
1. Statutory notification of disease (e.g. poliomyelitis)
2. Registrable diseases (e.g. cancer)
3. Surveys

## TYPES OF EPIDEMIOLOGICAL SURVEYS

1. Descriptive studies (typically measure incidence or prevalence of disease) may be:
   (i) *Cross-sectional,* e.g. comparison of severity of periodontal disease in individuals of different ages at a single point of time
   (ii) *Longitudinal,* e.g. measure progress of periodontal disease followed in the *same* individuals as age advances
2. Analytical studies (test associations between disease prevalence and hypothetical causative factors)
   (i) Cohort studies. Test changes in prevalence in those exposed with those not exposed (cohort = group subject to a common environmental influence *or* group sharing same year of birth) e.g. longitudinal study on prevalence of caries developing in fluoride and non-fluoride communities
   (ii) Case/control studies. e.g. retrospective study of degree of exposure to fluorides in caries-active and caries-free patients
3. Experimental studies — test effect of hypothetical causative factors, e.g. by increasing level of fluoride intake in one group and comparing amount of caries developing in controls with low fluoride intake

## PROBLEMS AFFECTING ACCURACY OF STUDIES

1. Defining observation to be made, e.g. how to define the 'fit' of dentures
2. Accuracy of observation, e.g. how to assess oral hygiene or severity of gingivitis objectively
3. Practical limitations, e.g. radiographic equipment necessary for early interstitial caries or periodontal bone loss
4. Inter-observer variation — especially with indices of periodontal disease

## EXAMPLES OF VARIABLES SUSCEPTIBLE TO EPIDEMIOLOGICAL INVESTIGATION WHICH MAY AFFECT DENTAL DISEASE

1. Age, e.g. increasing periodontal destruction or decreasing severity of caries with age (e.g. due to loss of teeth or changes in eating habits)
2. Sex, e.g. women may have better oral hygiene (possibly for cosmetic reasons or because of greater concern about loss of teeth)
3. Socioeconomic status — has important associations with dental state and generally interrelated with:
   (i) Type of occupation
   (ii) Educational levels
   (iii) Knowledge about causes and prevention of dental disease
   (iv) Individuals' level of knowledge about their own or children's state of dental health
   (v) Attitudes towards preservation of teeth and dental treatment
   (vi) Patterns of dental attendance
   (vii) Levels of oral hygiene

## EXAMPLES OF EPIDEMIOLOGICAL FINDINGS RELATING TO DENTAL CARIES

1. Low caries prevalence with traditional ('primitive') diets containing little sugar (e.g. Eskimo)
2. Increased caries prevalence associated with change from 'primitive' (low sugar diet) to Westernised, high sugar diet
3. Increasing prevalence of caries associated with increasing sugar intake in Westernised countries (since approx. 1860)
4. Fall in caries prevalence associated with decreased sugar consumption in World War II
5. Low caries associated with low sugar intake in patients with hereditary fructose intolerance
6. Lack of evidence of association of dental caries with malnutrition
7. Low caries prevalence associated with fluoride in water over 1 ppm (e.g. Maldon, Essex)
8. Reduction in caries prevalence compared with control areas after fluoridation of water (e.g. Kingston and Newburgh)
9. Reduced caries prevalence associated with increased molybdenum intake (e.g. Hungary, New Zealand)
10. Increased caries prevalence associated with increased selenium intake (e.g. Oregon)
11. Some association between oral *Strep. mutans* and early caries activity, but also conflicting findings
12. Decreasing caries prevalence in children in Britain and some other countries

## EXAMPLES OF EPIDEMIOLOGICAL FINDINGS RELATING TO PERIODONTAL DISEASE

1. Prevalence of gingivitis and periodontal destruction age-related
    (i) Onset of gingivitis typically detected at age 5 or earlier
    (ii) Pocketing. Detectable in about 1 per cent at age 10 and in about 10 per cent at age 20
2. Sex. Periodontal disease generally more prevalent and severe in males but earlier total tooth loss in females
3. Socioeconomic status. More severe periodontal disease and earlier tooth loss in lower income and lower education groups
4. Oral hygiene. Close relationship between level of oral hygiene and prevalence and severity of gingivitis
5. General relationship between oral hygiene levels and severity of periodontal destruction but association less close than with gingivitis — some conflicting findings
6. No consistent relationship between level of nutrition and periodontal disease
7. Relationship between fluoride intake and periodontal disease — conflicting findings
*Note*: Figures for prevalence and severity of gingivitis and periodontal destruction vary in different surveys due to lack of objective means of quantifying oral hygiene or severity of disease

## EPIDEMIOLOGY OF CANCER OF THE LIP AND MOUTH

1. Age incidence: 98 per cent of cases over 40
2. Overall incidence about 1 per 20 000 of the population: increases to about 1 per 1000 after age 75
3. More common in males (about 2 to 1 in 1950s) but declining in males and sex incidence almost equal in SE England
4. Lip cancer rare in women
5. Site. Tongue most common intra-oral site (but lip more common than tongue)
6. Over 90 per cent are squamous cell carcinomas
7. Wide international variation in incidence and of aetiological factors
8. No quantitive relation between smoking or alcohol consumption and mouth cancer in Britain — *increased* smoking and drinking of past decades associated with *declining* oral cancer rates
9. 5-year survival rates
   (i) Lip — about 90 per cent
   (ii) Intra-oral — between about 40 and 50 per cent
10. Survival rates dependent on
    (i) Age — deteriorating survival with increasing age
    (ii) Sex — better survival rates in women
    (iii) Site — the further back the growth the worse the prognosis
    (iv) Quality of treatment

## APPENDIX: INDICES OF DENTAL DISEASE

### DENTAL CARIES
1. DMF. Widely used but takes no account of natural shedding of deciduous teeth or of losses due to periodontal disease
2. DMFS. Measures new points of attack on same tooth. Therefore more sensitive index of severity but needs radiographs to detect early interstitial lesions

### PERIODONTAL DISEASE

**Variables usually measured**
1. Amount of plaque and calculus
2. Extent of gingivitis and pocketing
3. Severity of gingival bleeding
4. Amount of alveolar bone loss

*Note*: These assessments are not objective

## THE PLAQUE INDEX
0 = Absent
1 = Plaque adhering to gingival margin and adjacent tooth surface
2 = Moderate accumulation of plaque within gingival pocket, on the margin and/or adjacent tooth
3 = Abundant plaque within gingival pocket and/or gingival margin and adjacent tooth

## THE ORAL HYGIENE INDEX (SIMPLIFIED)
Six tooth surfaces usually chosen. Each surface scored for plaque and calculus*

### Plaque
0 = Absent
1 = Covering not more than one-third of tooth
2 = Covering more than one-third but less than two-thirds of tooth
3 = Covering more than two-thirds of tooth

### Calculus
0 = Absent
1 = Supragingival calculus covering not more than one-third of tooth
2 = Supragingival calculus covering more than one-third but not more than two-thirds of tooth, or flecks of subgingival calculus round necks of teeth, or both
3 = Supragingival calculus covering more than two-thirds of tooth or continuous heavy band of subgingival calculus round neck of tooth, or both

The mean plaque score and the mean calculus score added to give Oral Hygiene Index*

*Note*: A *high* Oral Hygiene score indicates severe oral *neglect* (confusing — is it not?)

## THE GINGIVAL INDEX
Circumference of gingival margin divided into four (mesial, distal, buccal and lingual) and each scored
0 = Normal gingiva
1 = Mild inflammation; slight change in colour, slight oedema, no bleeding on probing
2 = Moderate inflammation, redness, oedema and glazing; bleeding on probing
3 = Severe inflammation, severe redness and oedema; ulceration; spontaneous bleeding

The score for each area is totalled and sum divided by 4 to provide gingival index for whole mouth*

THE PERIODONTAL INDEX

0 = No overt inflammation or loss of function due to destruction of supporting tissues

1 = Mild gingivitis. Inflammation of gingival margin but this does not surround tooth

2 = Gingivitis. Inflammation surrounds tooth but no detectable break in epithelial attachment

3 = Gingivitis with pocket formation. True pocketing but no mobility, migration or interference with function

The Periodontal Index is sum of scores for individual teeth divided by number of teeth examined*

* The mathematical manipulation of these 'scores' is meaningless since they are not measurements but arbitrary figures given to subjective assessments

# Pathological aspects of dental extractions

LOCAL COMPLICATIONS
1. Fractured roots
2. Infection (dry socket or osteomyelitis)
3. Haemorrhage
4. Fracture of jaw
5. Injury to soft tissues
6. Involvement of antrum
7. Fracture of tuberosity
8. Delayed healing

SYSTEMIC COMPLICATIONS
1. Infective endocarditis
2. Inhalation of tooth (respiratory obstruction or lung abscess)

## HEALING OF SOCKETS

1. Bleeding into socket
2. Organisation of clot
3. Epithelialisation of surface
4. Woven bone formation
5. Resorption of lamina dura
6. Replacement by lamellar bone
7. Remodelling of alveolar ridge

## DELAYED HEALING OF SOCKETS

1. Infection
2. Persistent haemorrhage
3. Oro-antral fistula
4. Neoplasm
5. Irradiation
6. Corticosteroid and/or cytotoxic treatment
7. Scurvy

## DRY SOCKET

### Possible causative factors
1. Local ischaemia
   (i) Lower molars
   (ii) Excessive local anaesthetic
   (iii) Osteosclerosis (e.g. Paget's disease)
   (iv) Radiotherapy

2. Excessive trauma
3. Excessive tissue fibrinolytic activity
4. Infection by fibrinolytic bacteria
5. Unknown factors

### Pathology
Localised osteitis of socket wall with gradual sequestration.
Healing by granulation from the base

### Diagnosis
1. Severe aching pain after extraction
2. Socket empty of clot
3. Bare bone of socket lining visible
4. Small sequestra later exfoliated
5. Healing by granulation from depths of socket — hastened by
   repeated irrigation and dressings to exclude food debris

## HAEMORRHAGE

### Local factors
1. Excessive trauma
2. Damage to blood vessel
3. Infection (secondary haemorrhage? ever)

### Systemic factors
1. Purpura
2. Clotting defects (p. 108)

## COMPLICATIONS INVOLVING THE ANTRUM

1. Displacement of root into antrum
2. Oro-antral fistula
3. Avulsion of tuberosity

### Root in antrum — contributory causes
1. Low antral floor
2. Attempting to dig molar root out via socket

**Diagnosis**
1. Disappearance of root
2. Signs of fistula (see below)
3. Sinusitis
4. Root in antrum in radiographs

**Management**
1. Explain to patient
2. Radiographs
   (i) Root in antrum, *or*
   (ii) Root between lining and floor?
3. Remove root via adequate muco-periosteal flap, *or*
4. Keep under observation if root outside lining
5. Give decongestants (ephedrine nasal drops; tinct. benzoin Co. inhalations)
6. Give systemic antibiotic (usually penicillin)

## ORO-ANTRAL FISTULA

**Predisposing factors**
1. Inadequate bone around tooth
   (i) Low antral floor
   (ii) Periodontal or periapical destruction
   (iii) Isolated tooth
2. Excessive trauma

**Diagnosis**
1. Air entering mouth during swallowing
2. Blood or other fluids entering nose
3. Frothing from socket
4. Air forced into mouth when blowing nose later
5. Salty or septic taste
6. Swelling from socket (prolapse of antral polyp)

**Management**
1. Close with muco-periosteal flap
2. If very small, cover with acrylic plate; may heal
3. Suture Whitehead's varnish pack over opening — may heal or can be repaired later
4. Give antibiotic (usually penicillin)

**Established infected fistula**
1. Treat sinusitis
2. Give course of antibiotic
3. Give decongestants
4. Remove any polyps via antral window
5. Close with muco-periosteal flap

## AVULSION OF TUBEROSITY

1. Isolated molars
2. Low antral floor

### Effects
1. Oro-antral fistula
2. Impaired denture retention

### Management
Suture opening and cover with acrylic plate

## MALERUPTED THIRD MOLARS

### Complications (indications for extraction)
1. Pain
1. Pericoronitis
3. Caries
4. Damage to second molar
5. Cyst formation
6. Eruption under denture

## PERICORONITIS

### Causes
1. Stagnation under gum flap of partially erupted $\overline{8}$
2. Accumulation of plaque and food debris
3. Biting on gum flap
4. Spread of ulcerative gingivitis (rarely)

### Diagnosis
1. Pain
2. Swelling round partially erupted $\overline{8}$
3. Limited opening

### Management
1. Irrigate under flap
2. Frequent hot mouth washes
3. Give penicillin or metronidazole if severe
4. Remove tooth biting on flap if appropriate
5. Radiographs for position of $\overline{8}$
6. Remove lower molar (if appropriate) in quiescent phase

## MALERUPTED UPPER CANINES

### Complications
1. Orthodontic problems
2. Resorption of teeth
3. Cyst formation
4. Eruption under denture

### Management
1. Leave (if possible) *or*
2. Extract, *or*
3. Bring back into arch (if space available) by traction *or*
4. Transplant into previously prepared socket. Splint. Do *not* root fill before transplantation

# Severe infections

## ACUTE OSTEOMYELITIS OF JAWS

1. Rare
2. Infection usually dental, i.e. anaerobes or gram-negative aerobic bacteria
3. Sources of infection — dental abscess, fracture through periodontal pocket, penetrating wound, open fracture
4. Pathology
   (i) Spread of infection in medullary spaces, suppuration
   (ii) Thromboses of intra-bony vessels, necrosis of bone recognisable by absence of osteocytes
   (iii) Stretching of periosteum and peripheral new bone formation
   (iv) Osteoclastic separation of sequestra. Healing by granulation and woven bone formation

**Diagnosis and management**
1. Mandible, mainly adult males
2. (i) Severe aching pain, swelling (oedema and periosteal expansion)
   (ii) Gums red and swollen, teeth loosened
   (iii) Anaesthesia of lip
   (iv) Trismus, regional lymphadenopathy
3. Systemic effects usually slight. Sometimes fever and malaise in acute phase
4. Irregular moth-eaten areas of radiolucency after about 10 days. Sequestra more radiopaque. New bone formation, especially along lower border, later
5. Obtain pus for microbiology
6. Give penicillin 600 mg (i.m. 4 times daily by injection) or other antibiotic if sensitivity tests dictate
7. Drain exudate. Remove sequestra when separated

## POST-IRRADIATION OSTEOMYELITIS

1. Severe ischaemia of bone due to obliterative endarteritis
2. Infection (e.g. after extraction) can lead to intractable osteomyelitis of ischaemic area
3. Mucosa and skin may break down, exposing necrotic area of jaw
4. Prevention — clear all unhealthy teeth before irradiation or ensure (if patient anxious to retain natural teeth) that everything to minimise risk of extraction in future
5. If apical periodontitis develops or periodontal bone loss severe after radiotherapy, temporise by giving antibiotics to avoid extractions
6. If osteomyelitis develops, give massive doses of antibiotics. In severe cases resect affected area at safe distance from ischaemic area. (See also management of xerostomia)

## CELLULITIS

1. Rare
2. Anaerobic or ß haemolytic streptococcal infection
3. Spread of infection along fascial spaces, especially from lingual molar region below mylohyoid line into sublingual and/or submandibular spaces
4. Medial pterygoid space infection typically due to infected needle or local anaesthetic
5. Give penicillin 600 mg 4 times daily i.m. (or other antibiotic if tests dictate)

## LUDWIG'S ANGINA

1. Rare
2. Severe cellulitis of sublingual and submandibular spaces spreading to parapharyngeal space
3. Board-like swelling of soft tissues of floor of mouth, base of tongue, front of neck, spreading down side of neck
4. Fever and severe malaise. Respiratory obstruction by tongue pushed into pharynx, or oedema of glottis
5. Incise front of neck to relieve pressure. Give penicillin initially (see above). Intubate or tracheostomy if necessary
6. Complications — can be fatal from asphyxia or acute mediastinitis

## ACTINOMYCOSIS

1. Cause — usually *Actinomyces israelii* from mouth
2. May follow extraction or fracture, but pathogenesis unknown
3. (i) Infection spreads through soft tissues near angle of jaw
   (ii) Clumps of actinomyces (sulphur granules) surrounded by polymorphs with peripheral lymphocytes and fibrous wall
   (iii) Multiple abscesses and skin sinuses eventually form suppurating, fibrotic, honeycomb mass

### Diagnosis and management

1. Mainly adult males — typically otherwise healthy. Little pain; firm, nodular swelling with suppuration and puckering and pigmentation of skin, spreading down side of neck
2. Obtain pus for anaerobic culture. (Positive results likely only if sulphur granules present)
3. Give penicillin (or tetracycline) for several weeks
4. Drain adequately

# Cysts of the jaws

1. General mechanism of formation
   (i) Epithelial proliferation
   (ii) Central fluid accumulation — increasing hydrostatic pressure
   (iii) Resorption of surrounding bone
2. Commonest chronic swellings of the jaws
3. Most are odontogenic
4. General diagnostic features (with rare exceptions):
   (i) Usually related to a tooth
   (ii) Slow, painless expansive growth
   (iii) Sharply defined, rounded radiolucency
   (iv) Displacement of adjacent teeth
   (v) Respond to enucleation (but always biopsy to confirm diagnosis)
5. Differential diagnosis — see Tables 1 and 2

**Table 1** Important radiolucent (cyst-like) lesions of jaws

| | |
|---|---|
| 1. Cysts | Odontogenic |
| | Non-odontogenic |
| 2. Tumours | Odontogenic |
| | Non-odontogenic (including metastatic) |
| 3. Tumour-like lesions | Giant cell granuloma |
| 4. Hyperparathyroidism (Osteitis fibrosa cystica) | |
| 5. Cherubism | |
| 6. Stafne bone cavity | |

**Table 2** Typical radiological characteristics of cysts and cyst-like lesions of jaws

| Monocular | Multilocular or pseudoloculated | Multiple lesions |
|---|---|---|
| Periodontal | Primordial | Hyperparathyroidism |
| Residual | Ameloblastoma | Jaw cyst, basal cell |
| Dentigerous | Giant cell | carcinoma syndrome |
| | granuloma | Metastases |
| 'Fissural' | Hyperparathyroidism | Multiple myeloma |
| Intra-osseous tumours | Cherubism | Cherubism |
| | (symmetrical) | |
| Metastases | Myxoma | |
| (ragged outline) | | |
| Stafne bone cavity | | |

*Note*: Diagnosis of cysts usually made on clinical and radiological features but confirmation of diagnosis depends on histopathology

## CLASSIFICATION

### CYSTS WITH EPITHELIAL LINING

**Odontogenic cysts**
1. Periodontal (apical, lateral or residual)
2. Dentigerous
3. Primordial
4. Calcifying odontogenic cyst
5. Cysts within a neoplasm

**Non-odontogenic (so-called fissural) cysts**
1. Nasopalatine, median palatine, etc.
2. Nasolabial

**Cysts of doubtful origin**
Globulomaxillary

### CYSTS WITHOUT EPITHELIAL LINING (NON-ODONTOGENIC)
1. Solitary (simple) bone cysts
2. Aneurysmal bone cyst

**Miscellaneous**
Stafne bone cavity

## ODONTOGENIC CYSTS

### PERIODONTAL (RADICULAR) CYSTS
1. Chronic periapical inflammation, proliferation of granulation tissue and epithelial rests of Malassez
2. Squamous epithelial lining; hyperplastic, thin and flattened, or destroyed. Chronic inflammation; sometimes clefts
3. Form nearly 70 per cent of all jaw cysts
4. Form at apex of dead tooth (clinical features — see above)
5. Management. Up to 2 cm in diameter — usually resolve after endodontic treatment. Otherwise enucleate. Marsupialisation rarely necessary.
6. Biopsy lining to confirm diagnosis
7. Extract or root fill affected tooth

### RESIDUAL CYST
Periodontal cyst remaining after extraction of causative tooth (features and management as above)

### LATERAL CYST
Cyst from lateral branch of root canal or rarely secondary to inflammation in periodontal pocket

### DENTIGEROUS CYSTS
1. Cystic change between layers of reduced enamel epithelium after formation of enamel
2. Cyst surrounds crown; attached to neck of tooth
3. Squamous epithelium lining, inflammation may be absent

**Diagnosis**
1. Upper 3s and lower 8s most often affected
2. Most common jaw cyst in children but overall more common in adults
3. Radiology: cyst surrounds crown of displaced buried tooth
4. Enucleate or marsupialise — occasionally a 3 can be brought back into the arch, or transplanted
5. Biopsy lining

### ERUPTION CYSTS
1. Superficial, overlying crown of tooth
2. Probably type of dentigerous cyst
3. Tense dark blue swelling, typically over molars in infants
4. No bone resorption
5. Probably rupture spontaneously but, if necessary, excise

## PRIMORDIAL CYSTS ('ODONTOGENIC KERATOCYSTS')

1. Cystic change in enamel organ or dental primordium — tooth typically missing
2. Well-formed squamous epithelial lining, uniform thickness, well-defined basal cell layer. Variable keratin formation. Inflammation normally absent. Lining much folded
3. Budding from deep surface of lining or daughter cyst formation occasionally
4. Growth infiltrative rather than expansive

### Diagnosis

1. Typically, multiloculated appearance in radiographs
2. Extent of cyst typically greater than clinical swelling
3. Enucleate
4. Biopsy lining
5. Recurrence common, sometimes after 10 or more years. Follow up

## ODONTOGENIC KERATOCYST

Literally, cyst of odontogenic origin with keratin formation. e.g. a primordial cyst, but only a minority of primordial cysts form orthokeratin while other cysts may. Confusing term. Risk of recurrence NOT related to presence of keratin but to *type of lining*

## CYSTS IN TUMOURS

1. Most often in ameloblastoma
2. Radiologically may mimic periodontal or dentigerous cyst
3. Extensive cyst formation flattens epithelial lining — also mimicking simple cyst
4. Tumour may form only restricted area of mural thickening
5. Examine cyst linings thoroughly histologically

## CALCIFYING ODONTOGENIC CYST

1.  (i) Epithelium may resemble ameloblastoma or be squamous in type
    (ii) Pale areas of abnormal keratinisation, outlines of cells with nuclear holes (ghost cells)
    (iii) Ghost cells may fill cyst cavity or provoke foreign body reaction
    (iv) Ghost cells may calcify
    (v) Not always cystic. May be a benign tumour

### Diagnosis

1. Typically in mandible. No special age or sex predominance. Rare
2. Behaves clinically like a cyst
3. Radiolucent area, occasionally flecks of calcification
4. Occasionally in soft tissues
5. May be associated with tooth, denticle or odontome
6. Enucleate; unlikely to recur
7. Diagnosis confirmed by biopsy

## NEOPLASTIC CHANGE IN CYSTS
1. Carcinomatous change in simple cysts *possible*, but rare — an almost insignificant hazard
2. Diagnosis; neoplastic change suggested by onset of
   (i) Pain
   (ii) Paraesthesia of lip
   (iii) Increased rate of growth
   (iv) Ragged radiological outline
3. Confirm by biopsy

## NON-ODONTOGENIC CYSTS

### NASOPALATINE (INCISIVE CANAL) CYST
1. From remnants of nasopalatine duct
2. Lining — squamous and/or ciliated columnar (respiratory) epithelium
3. Vessels and nerves (canal contents) associated

#### Diagnosis
1. Midline swelling in anterior palate. (Median palatine, median alveolar and incisive papilla cysts probably not distinct entities)
2. Round or heart-shaped radiolucency
3. Enucleate. Other remnants of duct lining may cause recurrence
4. Histological features in biopsy

#### 'FISSURAL' CYSTS
1. Development of face by fusion of embryonic processes no longer accepted
2. 'Globulo-maxillary' and other putative fissural cysts in anterior maxilla probably odontogenic
3. Enucleate

### NASOLABIAL CYST
1. Forms in soft tissue deep to and filling out nasolabial groove
2. Aetiology unknown

## CYSTS WITHOUT EPITHELIAL LINING (NON-ODONTOGENIC)

### SOLITARY BONE CYST
1. Aetiology unknown. No evidence of traumatic or haemorrhagic origin
2. Bony walls with thin fibrous lining or bare
3. Serous or bloodstained fluid or empty interior

**Diagnosis**
1. Typically radiolucent area, arching up between roots of teeth, but little expansion. Outline less sharp than true cysts
2. Females more frequently affected, usually before age 25
3. Treatment. Opening bone cavity and (if necessary) curretting wall leads to healing
4. Biopsy any tissue lining cavity

ANEURYSMAL BONE CYST
1. Bone cavity filled with highly vascular connective tissue resembling blood-filled sponge. Haemorrhages and giant cells
2. Possibly developmental anomaly

**Diagnosis**
1. Usually seen before age 25. Swelling sometimes expansive
2. Radiology: unilocular, trabeculated or soap-bubble area of lucency
3. Enucleate
4. Confirm by biopsy

## COMPLICATIONS OF CYSTS

1. Infection
2. Fracture of mandible

## STAFNE BONE CAVITY

1. Deep, rounded depression of lingual plate of mandible filled with salivary tissue
2. Mandible, near lower border and angle. Asymptomatic
3. Adults; very rare in children
4. Cyst-like area of radiolucency but static
5. Explore if any doubt as to diagnosis

# Tumours and tumour-like lesions of the jaws

1. Odontogenic tumours
2. Primary bone tumours
3. Secondary (metastatic) tumours
4. Lymphoreticular tumours
5. Histiocytosis X

ODONTOGENIC TUMOURS

**Epithelial**
1. Ameloblastoma
2. Adenomatoid odontogenic tumour ('adeno-ameloblastoma')
3. Calcifying epithelial odontogenic tumour

**Connective tissue**
1. Cementomas and cemental dysplasias
2. Odontogenic fibroma
3. Myxoma

**Mixed**
1. Ameloblastic fibroma
2. Odontomes (usually hamartomas)

NON-ODONTOGENIC TUMOURS
Melanotic neuroectodermal tumour of infancy

PRIMARY BONE TUMOURS

**Benign**
1. Fibroma — ossifying and non-ossifying
2. Chondroma
3. Osteoma
4. Central giant cell granuloma
5. From any other connective tissue structure

**Malignant**
1. Osteosarcoma
2. Fibrosarcoma
3. Chondrosarcoma
4. From any other connective tissue structure

SECONDARY (METASTATIC) TUMOURS
Carcinomas

LYMPHORETICULAR TUMOURS OF BONE
1. Multiple myeloma and solitary plasmacytoma
2. Histiocytic lymphoma ('reticulum cell sarcoma')
3. Burkitt's lymphoma
4. Ewing's tumour

## ODONTOGENIC TUMOURS

AMELOBLASTOMA
1. Typically, processes of ameloblast-like cells surrounding loosely
   arranged stellate cells with microscopic or gross cyst formation.
   Variable squamous metaplasia
2. Slowly invasive mainly into cancellous spaces
3. Non-metastasising

**Diagnosis**
1. Clinically 80 per cent in posterior mandible or ramus. Mainly
   males over 40
2. Slow growing, painless swelling. Can involve soft tissue
3. Typically, multilocular cyst on radiographs. Can mimic
   periodontal or dentigerous cysts occasionally
4. Confirm diagnosis by biopsy. Excise widely. Preferably leave
   lower border of jaw intact. Follow up and re-operate if necessary.

ADENOMATOID ODONTOGENIC TUMOUR
1. Whorls of epithelium, microcysts lined by columnar epithelium,
   amorphous or cystalline calcifications. Fibrous capsule
2. Surrounds or contiguous with tooth.

**Diagnosis**
1. Late teens or young adults, especially females
2. Slow-growing swelling or 'cyst' on radiograph, usually anterior
   maxilla
3. Enucleate. No tendency to recur
4. Confirm diagnosis by biopsy

## CALCIFYING EPITHELIAL ODONTOGENIC TUMOUR (CEOT; PINDBORG TUMOUR)

1. 'Polyhedral' squamous epithelial cells, gross nuclear pleomorphism (simulating carcinoma), amyloid, rounded or confluent calcifications
2. Locally invasive

### Diagnosis

1. Mainly adults. Usually mandible
2. Slow-growing painless swelling
3. Radiolucent area with variable areas of radiopacity. Poorly defined margins
4. Diagnosis by biopsy. Excise widely. Follow up. May recur

## CALCIFYING ODONTOGENIC CYST
(See p. 50)

## CEMENTOMAS AND CEMENTAL DYSPLASIAS

### Benign cementoblastoma

1. Irregular or rounded mass of cementum attached to tooth root. Pagetoid ('mosaic') pattern of reversal lines. Peripheral zone of uncalcified precementum and fibrous pericementum
2. Probably a benign tumour
3. Usually males under 25
4. Radiopaque periapical mass with lucent border in molar region
5. Enucleate

### Cementifying fibroma

1. Rounded mass of connective tissue containing enlarging nodules of cementum, finally forming densely calcified mass
2. Mostly in middle-aged. Usually mandibular molars
3. Rounded periapical area of radiolucency (but teeth vital). Often increasing calcification until completely radiopaque and stationary

### Periapical cemental dysplasia

1. Essentially similar to cementifying fibroma
2. Mainly women after middle age. Usually lower incisor region. Periapical radiolucency initially but teeth vital. Increasing calcification

### Gigantiform cementoma

1. Rounded masses resembling secondary cementum
2. Usually middle-aged black women
3. Multiple radiopaque masses near apices especially of molars, often symmetrical. Rarely, expansion of jaw

## ODONTOGENIC FIBROMA
1. Circumscribed cellular fibrous mass containing epithelial rests adjacent to a tooth
2. Symptomless cyst-like or multilocular radiolucency
3. May contain calcifications

## MYXOMA
1. Scanty spindle or stellate cells with fine fibrils in loose mucoid stroma sometimes containing epithelial rests. Typically widespread infiltration of bone
2. Mainly young adults. Usually painless swelling
3. Radiolucent area with soap-bubble appearance
4. Recurrence frequent in spite of wide excision. May persist (inactively) for many years.

## AMELOBLASTIC FIBROMA
1. Proliferating enamel organ-like epithelium in dentine papilla-like mesenchyme. Both elements may be neoplastic. Non-infiltrative
2. Clinically and radiologically resembles ameloblastoma but enucleated readily
3. Exceedingly rare

## MALIGNANT ODONTOGENIC TUMOURS
1. Malignant counterparts of odontogenic tumours reported
2. All exceedingly rare
3. Diagnosis confirmed histologically, as with all other tumours

## ODONTOMES
1. Malformations (hamartomas) of dental hard tissues. Range from minor morphological anomalies to gross disorganisation of development
2. Classification
   a. Enameloma (enamel pearl)
   b. Dentinoma
   c. Cementomas (see above)
   d. Composite
      (i) Compound — multiple small tooth-like denticles
      (ii) Complex — irregular, cauliflower-like mass of dentine, enamel and cementum with central branched pulp
   (*Note:* Despite grossly irregular morphology, dental hard tissues maintain normal relationship to one another)
3. Typically behave like teeth, i.e. cease growth after completion of development and tend to erupt
4. Occasionally behave as tumours (e.g. cementoblastoma) or associated with neoplasms, e.g. ameloblastoma

## NON-ODONTOGENIC TUMOURS

### MELANOTIC (NEUROECTODERMAL) JAW TUMOUR OF INFANCY ('MELANO AMELOBLASTOMA', PROGONOMA)

1. Probably originates from neural crest
2. Pigmented (melanin-containing) cells with pale nuclei surround clefts or small spaces. Non-pigmented cells with large pale nuclei in small groups or surrounded by pigmented cells. Connective tissue stroma forms most of mass
3. Infants, usually 3 months old or less; females predominantly
4. Typically maxilla. Rate of growth variable
5. Radiolucent area. Outline cyst-like or ragged
6. Unlikely to recur after excision

## PRIMARY BENIGN OSSEOUS TUMOURS OF THE JAWS

### FIBROMA

1. Whorls of collagen fibres and fibroblasts
2. Periosteal superficial firm swelling or endosteal rounded radiolucency and slow expansion
3. Excise or enucleate

### OSSIFYING FIBROMA

1. Cellular fibrous tissue containing globular calcified bodies (not distinguishable from cementifying fibroma)
2. Usually mandible in young adults
3. Slow-growing painless swelling. Circumscribed radiolucency, speckled calcifications. Progressive radiopacity
4. Excise (unlikely to recur)

### CHONDROMA

1. Cartilage containing small chondrocytes. Variable calcification. All gradations to chondrosarcoma
2. Any age. Painless slow-growing swelling
3. Irregular radiolucent area with variable radiopacities.
4. Excise widely — may prove to be sarcomatous despite microscopic apperance

### OSTEOMA

1. (i) Compact. Lamellae of dense bone, few osteocytes
   (ii) Cancellous. Bony trabeculae with lamellated cortex
2. Mainly young adults. Painless, very slow-growing. Endosteal or periosteal. Radiological features accordingly
3. Excise if causing inconvenience

## TORI

1. (i) Torus palatinus — centre of midline of palate. Hard, rounded, sometimes grooved
   (ii) Torus mandibularis — lingually, beside premolars, symmetrical
2. Very slow-growing. Usually noticed in middle age
3. Excise if affecting denture fit

## CENTRAL GIANT CELL GRANULOMA OF THE JAWS

1. Multinucleate osteoclast-like cells in vascular spindle cell stroma
2. Usually before age 20, females more than males. Usually mandible
3. Painless swelling. Occasionally rapid growth and pain
4. Rounded radiolucency, not sharply defined, faint 'loculation'
5. Biopsy. Blood chemistry to exclude hyperparathyroidism
6. Curette. Repeat if residual areas persist. Wide excision unnecessary — not a neoplasm

## OSTEOCLASTOMA (GIANT CELL TUMOUR OF BONE)

Probably does not affect jaws. Aggressively destructive neoplasm

## PRIMARY MALIGNANT TUMOURS

### OSTEOSARCOMA

1. Occasionally post-irradiation. Rarely a complication of Paget's disease (but not in jaws)
2. Pleomorphic picture of dark, angular neoplastic osteoblasts, osteoid, bone, vascular fibrous tissue, cartilage and giant cells, irregularly associated
3. Most common *primary* malignant tumour of bone
4. Usually mandible in males age about 30
5. Painful swelling, rapid growth. Distortion of alveolus Paraesthesia or anaesthesia. Loosening of teeth. Bleeding
6. Completely irregular pattern of radiolucency and radiopacity. May be predominantly osteolytic or sclerotic
7. Radical excision if localised, and chemotherapy. Metastases to lungs common

### FIBROSARCOMA

1. Occasionally periosteal, rarely endosteal
2. Histopathology, etc., see page 90

## CHONDROSARCOMA

1. Cellular cartilage, pleomorphic, sometimes multinucleate chondrocytes (all degrees of differentiation from chondroma)
2. Typically aggressively invasive, metastases usually late
3. Usually in mandible age 30 to 50
4. Expansile, painful, hard swelling
5. Radical excision but poor prognosis. Death usually from local spread

## SECONDARY TUMOURS OF JAWS

### CARCINOMAS

1. Particularly from bronchus, breast, prostate, kidney or thyroid
2. Pathology: that of primary adeno or squamous cell carcinoma
3. Initially painless. Increasing swelling, pain, loosening of teeth, anaesthesia of lip
4. Typically ragged, radiolucent area in jaw. Sometimes sclerotic (especially prostate)
5. Biopsy
6. General physical, radiological and other investigations to find primary tumour if not already apparent
7. Bone metastases usually in advanced disease and treatment only palliative

## LYMPHORETICULAR TUMOURS

### MULTIPLE MYELOMA

1. Multifocal proliferation of neoplastic plasma cells
2. Immunoglobulin (usually IgG) over-production (monoclonal); hypergammaglobulinaemia; sometimes Bence Jones proteinuria and amyloidosis
3. Middle age or later. Anaemia, infections, renal dysfunction, bleeding. Painful bone lesions late. Pathological fractures
4. Multiple punched out areas of radiolucency, especially skull
5. Biopsy, blood and urine protein analysis
6. Chemotherapy, but eventually fatal

### SOLITARY PLASMACYTOMA

1. Intra-bony or soft tissue tumour of plasma cells
2. Typically no hypergammaglobulinaemia
3. Males predominantly. Area of radiolucency in jaw or soft swelling. No lymph node involvement
4. Biopsy. Skeletal survey. Haematological examination
5. Long survival after excision and/or radiotherapy but usually ultimately becomes multifocal

## HISTIOCYTIC LYMPHOMA ('RETICULUM CELL SARCOMA')
1. Pleomorphic histiocyte-like cells but progenitor cell controversial. Abundant reticulin fibres
2. Rare. Usually in under 40s. Swelling of bone, sometimes painful. Diffuse area of radiolucency
3. Radiotherapy — good 5-year survival (better prognosis than soft tissue counterpart)

## BURKITT'S (AFRICAN) LYMPHOMA
1. Predominantly Central Africa in endemic areas of falciparum malaria. Association with Epstein-Barr virus (*not* proven cause)
2. Closely packed lymphoblasts and histiocytes with clear cytoplasm (starry night appearance)
3. Children, Jaw lesions often initial feature
4. Expansion and destruction of jaw, distortion of alveolus, loosening of teeth, proptosis, rupture into soft tissues. Diffuse areas of radiolucency
5. Wide and rapid involvement of other bones and soft tissues but rarely lymph nodes
6. Often unusually good response to chemotherapy, otherwise rapidly fatal

## EWING'S TUMOUR
1. Progenitor cell unknown. Uniform picture of large round lymphocyte-like cells but very rare
2. Typically in mandible in under 40s
3. Expansile and destructive swelling. Variable reactive bone formation and spread into soft tissues
4. Metastases to other bones and lungs. Often present at diagnosis
5. Poor response to radiotherapy, surgery or chemotherapy

## HISTIOCYTOSIS X
1. Eosinophilic granuloma
2. Hand-Schüller-Christian disease (multifocal eosinophilic granuloma)
3. Letterer-Siwe disease
4. Eosinophilic granuloma appears to arise from Langerhans (macrophage-like) cells. Cell of origin of Letterer-Siwe disease more doubtful

## EOSINOPHILIC GRANULOMA
1. Jaws relatively frequently affected, often severely
2. Foamy 'histiocytes' containing cholesterol, foci of eosinophils and necrosis
3. Young adults especially males
4. Tumour-like focus of bone destruction or severe periodontal destruction with gross gingival recession

5. Typically solitary lesion but confirm by skeletal survey
6. Should respond to currettage and, if necessary, chemotherapy
7. Good prognosis unless multifocal lesions develop (rare)

## HAND-SCHÜLLER-CHRISTIAN DISEASE
1. Classically, bone lesions, exophthalmos, diabetes insipidus (in only 25 per cent)
2. Microscopically similar to solitary eosinophilic granuloma
3. Mainly children, chronic course
4. Punched out bone lesions (especially of skull), periodontal destruction with red, spongy gingivae. Lymph nodes, spleen and liver sometimes involved with progressive systemic deterioration
5. Mortality about 30 per cent
6. Treatment. Corticosteroids and cytotoxic drugs possibly helpful

## LETTERER-SIWE DISEASE
1. Predominantly soft tissue deposits of poorly differentiated 'histiocytes' with some polymorphs. Possibly a lymphoma
2. Usually infants. Acute or subacute progress
3. Involvement of lymphoid tissue, liver and marrow. Anaemia, pancytopenia, fever and cachexia
4. Bone lesions, occasionally multiple ill-defined osteomyelitis-like areas of radiolucency
5. Jaws. Rarely, widespread destruction of alveolar bone with loosening and exfoliation of teeth
6. Treatment — chemotherapy. Usually fatal especially in infants

*Note:* All of the histiocytoses are rare but any, particularly eosinophilic granuloma, can cause gross periodontal destruction and jaw lesions can be an early feature. Diagnosis (as with tumours) depends on biopsy of lesion repeated if necessary.

# Genetic, metabolic and other bone diseases

## GENETIC
1. Osteogenesis imperfecta
2. Osteopetrosis
3. Achondroplasia
4. Cleidocranial dysplasia
5. Cherubism (familial fibrous dysplasia)

## METABOLIC AND ENDOCRINE
1. Rickets
2. Scurvy
3. Hyperparathyroidism (primary and secondary)
4. Hypoparathyroidism
5. Acromegaly

## UNKNOWN CAUSE
1. Osteoporosis of ageing
2. Paget's disease (osteitis deformans)
3. The fibrous dysplasias

## GENETIC BONE DISEASES

### OSTEOGENESIS IMPERFECTA
1. Autosomal dominant
2. Collagen defect, impaired matrix formation by osteoblasts. Long bones slender but normal epiphyses
3. Brittle long bones but rapid healing. Jaws rarely affected
4. Typically gross deformities, blue sclerae. Dentinogenesis imperfecta often associated

### OSTEOPETROSIS (MARBLE BONE DISEASE)
1. Probably autosomal recessive
2. Failure of normal remodelling, especially osteoclastic resorption of bone
3. Bone dense, thick but weak. Marrow cavities obliterated
4. Complications: anaemia, compression of cranial nerves (e.g. optic atrophy, facial palsy, deafness, trigeminal lesions), fractures osteomyelitis

## ACHONDROPLASIA
1. Autosomal dominant. Most common form of dwarfism
2. Defect or aplasia of zone of provisional calcification of epiphyses
3. Short bones. Premature fusion of bones of base of skull and retrusion of maxilla with dish-face appearance

## CLEIDOCRANIAL DYSPLASIA
See page 8

## CHERUBISM
See Fibrous dysplasias

## METABOLIC AND ENDOCRINE BONE DISEASES

## RICKETS
1. Vitamin D deficiency — (dietary or lack of sunlight)
2. Impaired calcification of osteoid, proliferation of epiphyseal cartilage, disorganisation of osteochondral junction
3. Bones weak and deformable. Muscle weakness
4. Teeth (severe cases only) wide zone of pre-and interglobular dentine. Enamel normal. No increased susceptibility to caries
5. Give vitamin D. Remedy diet

## SCURVY
1. Vitamin C deficiency
2. In infants, decreased osteoid formation but normal calcification
3. Purpura. Subperiosteal bleeding with calcification of haematoma
4. No dental defects

## HYPERPARATHYROIDISM (PRIMARY)
1. Adenoma in 80 per cent
2. Increased excretion of phosphate and increased reabsorption of calcium. Increased osteoclastic bone resorption
3. Bone lesions — now rare
    (i) Foci of resorption by osteoclasts producing
    (ii) Multiple 'cysts' (osteitis fibrosa cystica) on radiographs, or
    (iii) Sometimes, 'ground glass' resorption
    (iv) Loss of lamina dura
    (v) Resorption of terminal phalangeal tufts
    (vi) Bone pain, pathological fractures
4. Renal calcifications
5. Diagnosis. Histopathology (but indistinguishable from giant cell granuloma), skeletal survey and blood chemistry
6. Raised plasma calcium, parathormone (PTH) and alkaline phosphatase. Phosphate low or normal (see Table 3)
7. Complications. Cardiovascular disease (especially hypertension). Renal failure. Peptic ulcer
8. Treatment. Total or subtotal parathyroidectomy

## Secondary hyperparathyroidism
1. Complication of chronic renal failure (including graft rejection)
2. Other features as for primary hyperparathyroidism

**Table 3** Blood chemistry in bone diseases

| | Calcium | Phosphate | Alkaline Phosphatase | Acid Phosphatase |
|---|---|---|---|---|
| Normal | 2.10–2.60 mmol/l (8.5–10 mg/ 100 ml) | 0.8–1.5 mmol/l (2.5–45 mg/ 100 ml) | 7–105 u/l* (1–13 KA u) | less than 0.7 u/l |
| Rickets | Calcium x phosphorus product less than 2.5 (SI units) 0r 30 (mg/100 ml) | | Variably raised | Normal |
| Hyperpara-thyroidism | >2.8 mmol/l | Normal or low | > 105 u/l | Normal |
| Hypopara-thyroidism | <2.0 mmol/l | Variably raised | Normal | Normal |
| Paget's disease | Typically normal | | Up to 700 u/l (100 KA u) | Normal |
| Prostatic metastases | Normal | Normal | Raised (esp. with sclerotic lesions) | Raised |
| Factors for conversion to SI units | mg/100 ml = 4 mmol/l | mg/100 ml = 3.1 × mmol/l | 7.1 × KA u = u/l | None |

*Raised in children and over 60

## HYPOPARATHYROIDISM (IDIOPATHIC)
1. Sometimes organ-specific auto-immune
2. Onset 6 months to late childhood
3. Skeleton normal
4. Low plasma calcium and PTH
5. Epithelial defects associated. Enamel hypoplasia in early-onset cases
6. Some cases have candida-endocrinopathy syndrome (p. 81)

## ACROMEGALY
1. Hypersecretion of growth hormone (GH) by pituitary adenoma after puberty
2. (i) Gross prognathism and separation of teeth
   (ii) Enlarged tongue
   (iii) Coarse, thick facial features
   (iv) Large, broad, spade-like hands and feet
3. Complications: diabetes mellitus, visual defects, weakness
4. Distortion of pituitary fossa on radiographs. Raised plasma GH levels
5. Enucleation or irradiation of tumour
6. Surgery for prognathism

## BONE DISEASE OF UNKNOWN CAUSE

### OSTEOPOROSIS
1. Primary — unknown cause, invariable concomitant of ageing
   Secondary — corticosteroids; disuse (inactivity)
2. Generalised loss of bone tissue, increased radiolucency of skeleton
3. Onset after about age 35. Highly variable progress
4. More severe in women
5. Complications (late). Fracture of femur, collapse of vertebrae

### PAGET'S DISEASE
1. May affect 5 per cent of population over 55 in UK
2. Aetiology unknown. Viral?
3. Anarchic disorganisation of normal remodelling of bone
4. Many osteoclasts and osteoblasts. Irregular resorption and repair of bone. 'Mosaic' of basophil reversal lines
5. Bones enlarged, thick but weak
6. Pelvis, skull (calvarium), limbs mainly affected. Maxilla sometimes, mandible (alone) very rarely
7. Early, increased radiolucency and woolly texture. Later, increasing sclerosis
8. Maxilla (when affected) symmetrically enlarged. General thickening of alveolar ridge
9. Massive craggy hypercementosis (with mosaic pattern) of teeth. Extractions may cause haemorrhage or osteomyelitis
10. Complications (according to bones affected and severity): fractures, deformities, compression of cranial nerves, bone pain. Osteosarcoma rare. Virtually never in jaws. Cardiac failure
11. Blood chemistry — Alkaline phosphatase up to 100 KAu, (700 u/l) calcium and phosphorus typically normal
12. Calcitonin or diphosphonates often control symptoms or progress

## THE FIBROUS DYSPLASIAS
General features:
1. Foci of cellular fibrous tissue replace normal bone; variable numbers of giant cells
2. Alternating formation and resorption of fine trabeculae of woven bone but gradually increasing ossification
3. Lesions form rounded swellings
4. Typically stabilisation and arrest after completion of skeletal growth
5. No significant changes in blood chemistry

### Polyostotic fibrous dysplasia
1. Multiple lesions, sometimes painful
2. Jaw lesions (especially maxilla) in up to 30 per cent
3. Radiographs. Often multilocular cystic appearance
4. Mainly girls
5. Precocious puberty, skin pigmentation, occasionally other endocrinopathies may be associated (Albright's syndrome)
6. Rare

### Monostotic fibrous dysplasia
1. Usually maxilla. Painless rounded swelling
2. (i) Rounded radiolucency. Margins ill-defined
   (ii) Ground glass or finely stippled texture. Gradually increasing opacity
   (iii) Cosmetic surgical reduction; preferably later when inactive

### Cherubism
1. Autosomal dominant
2. Histologically loose vascular connective tissue with many giant cells
3. Symmetrical lesions at angles of mandibles and (severe cases) maxillae
4. Multilocular cystic appearance. Teeth sometimes displaced
5. Arrest or regression after puberty

*Note*: Not now regarded as a fibrous dysplasia

### Diagnosis of fibrous dysplasias
1. Biopsy alone not reliably diagnostic
2. Diagnosis depends on combination of
   (i) Clinical features
   (ii) Radiological appearances
   (iii) Histopathology
   (iv) Behaviour of lesion

# The temporomandibular joint and related tissues

**LIMITATION OF MOVEMENT ('TRISMUS')**

INTRA-ARTICULAR CAUSES
1. Dislocation
2. Intra-capsular fracture
3. Pyogenic or other arthritides
4. Ankylosis (after infection or fracture)

EXTRA-ARTICULAR CAUSES
1. Infection and inflammation near joint, e.g. pericoronitis or
   following mandibular block
2. Pain-dysfunction syndrome
3. Fracture of necks of condyles
4. Fibrosis, e.g. irradiation or burns
5. Tetanus
6. Tetany
7. Drugs — phenothiazines and metoclopramide (mouth usually
   fixed in semi-open posture)

*Note*: Most are rare except temporary inflammatory stiffness and
pain-dysfunction syndrome; limitation of movement often due to or
associated with pain

**PAIN**
1. Pain-dysfunction syndrome
2. Chronic arthritides
3. Pyogenic arthritis
4. Giant cell (temporal) arthritis

## PAIN-DYSFUNCTION SYNDROME
1. Neuromuscular dysfunction; painful spasm of masticatory muscles
2. No joint pathology
3. Disorders of occlusion — no proven aetiological significance
4. Young women mostly affected
5. Dull pain in masseter region especially on mastication, locking in open position, clicking of joint, irregular path of closure (in varying combinations)
6. Reassure. Bite-raising appliance with free sliding occlusion or muscle training exercises usually effective. Diazepam may help
7. In older patients especially depression may be main underlying factor

## FRACTURES AND DISLOCATION
1. Bilateral fractures of necks of condyles may be unnoticed except as anterior open bite and limited movement later
2. Dislocation (e.g. under anaesthesia). Fixed open bite. Treat immediately by downward and backward manual pressure on lower molars

## PYOGENIC ARTHRITIS
1. Gonococcal (polyarticular), staphylococcal, etc. Virtually non-existent now
2. Possible complication of untreated osteomyelitis, penetrating wound or haematogenous
3. Pain, local signs of acute inflammation, limited movement
4. Aspirate joint for pus for microbiological diagnosis and sensitivities

## RHEUMATOID ARTHRITIS
1. Radiological changes common in TMJ when disease widespread
2. Symptoms typically insignificant. Clicking or discomfort. Pain uncommon (p. 120)

## OSTEOARTHROSIS
1. Radiological finding in some elderly patients
2. Symptoms rare or minimal

## GIANT CELL ARTERITIS
Occasionally causes severe ischaemic muscle pain during mastication (p. 121)

TETANUS
1. Typically after penetrating wound contaminated with soil
2. Trismus — most common early sign, often with stiffness of neck or back
3. Risus sardonicus — spasm of facial muscles giving typical suffering expression (moderately severe cases)
4. Suspect tetanus when local causes for trismus (e.g. pericoronitis) absent, in patient with history of recent wound
5. Admit to Intensive Care. Give purified antitoxin (test for allergy). Debride wound and give penicillin. Control spasms with muscle relaxants and artificial respiration

TETANY
1. Alkalosis or low plasma ionised calcium level
2. Most often due to hysterical overbreathing (hyperventilation syndrome) and $CO_2$ washout; rarely, acute hypoparathyroidism or rickets
3. Hyper-reactivity of muscles, spasms from minor stimuli, e.g. trismus or spasm of facial muscles when facial nerve in front of ear tapped (Chvostek's sign), spasms of small muscles of hands or feet. Wheezing. Sometimes fainting
4. If overbreathing, use rebreathing bag to increase $CO_2$ intake. Reassure but admit to hospital for assessment
5. Manage anxiety on future occasions, e.g. with sedation

# Stomatitis and related diseases

## INFECTIVE

### VIRAL
1. Herpetic stomatitis
   Herpes labialis
2. Herpes zoster
3. Hand, foot and mouth disease
4. Herpangina
5. Infectious mononucleosis
6. Chickenpox
7. Measles

### FUNGAL
*Candida albicans* infections
1. Thrush
2. Angular stomatitis
3. Denture stomatitis
4. Candidal leukoplakia (p. 80)
5. Mucocutaneous candidosis syndromes (p. 80)

### BACTERIAL
1. Syphilis
2. Gonorrhoea
3. Tuberculosis

## IMMUNOLOGICALLY MEDIATED OR OF DUBIOUS AETIOLOGY

1. Aphthous stomatitis
2. Lichen planus
3. Pemphigus vulgaris
4. Mucous membrane pemphigoid
5. Bullous erythema multiforme (Stevens-Johnson syndrome)
6. Lupus erythematosus

## MUCOSAL REACTIONS TO DRUGS
1. Local
2. Systemically mediated

## CHRONIC KERATOSES (WHITE LESIONS, LEUKOPLAKIAS)
1. Developmental
2. Frictional
3. Smoker's keratosis
4. Syphilitic
5. Chronic candidosis
6. Lichen planus
7. Idiopathic
8. Dysplastic (dyskeratotic)
9. Early carcinoma
10. Skin grafts

## INFECTIVE

PRIMARY HERPETIC STOMATITIS
1. Cause: Herpes simplex type 1 (rarely type 2)
2. Viral damage to epithelial cells, vesiculation, destruction of epithelium
3. At one time, a disease of childhood, but adults increasingly affected
4. Domed vesicles and painful ulcers. Any part of mouth
5. Gingivitis with or without ulcers
6. Acute febrile illness. Cervical lymphadenopathy
7. Smear — ballooning degeneration of epithelial cells, giant cells and inclusion bodies

### Diagnosis and management
1. Diagnosis is usually on clinical picture
2. Confirmed by rising titre of complement-fixing antibodies
3. Topical idoxuridine or acyclovir may hasten resolution

HERPES LABIALIS (COLD SORE, FEVER BLISTERS)
1. Recurrences in 10 to 30 per cent after primary infection
2. Virus (in inactive form) in trigeminal ganglia
3. Typically precipitated by febrile illness, strong sunshine, etc.
4. Clusters of vesicles, exudation and crusting at mucocutaneous junction of lips
5. Early topical idoxuridine may help hasten resolution

## HERPES ZOSTER OF TRIGEMINAL AREA
1. Cause — varicella zoster virus. Reactivation of latent virus
2. Pathology as for herpes simplex. Posterior root ganglia also affected
3. Patients typically middle aged or over. May indicate immune defect, e.g. Hodgkin's disease
4.   (i) Burning sensations or toothache-like pain first
     (ii) Vesicular rash in sensory area of V
     (iii) Vesicular stomatitis in corresponding area of mucosa
5. Bed rest for severe cases. Some response to topical idoxuridine

**Diagnosis**
1. Clinical picture (as above)
2. Evidence of previous varicella (high titre of antibodies)
3. No method of serological diagnosis of zoster itself

## HAND, FOOT AND MOUTH DISEASE
1. Cause — coxsackie A viruses
2. Highly infective. Predominantly school children
3. Mild vesicular stomatitis. No gingivitis
4. Vesicular rash on extremities
5. No specific treatment

**Diagnosis**
1. Clinical picture usually characteristic
2. Culture of virus
3. Rising titre of antibodies

   *Note*: 2 and 3 rarely needed as disease mild and brief usually

## HERPANGINA
1. Cause — coxsackie A viruses
2. Minute vesicles, painful ulcers and erythema in oropharynx
3. Acute severe sore throat, dysphagia, fever and malaise
4. No specific treatment. Bed rest

## INFECTIOUS MONONUCLEOSIS
1. Cause — Epstein Barr virus
2. Mainly adolescents or young adults
3. Typically, sore throat, fever, lymphadenopathy
4. Petechiae and erythema of soft palate and pharynx. Sometimes oral ulceration
5. Cervical lymph nodes typically first affected
6. Anginose type — severe ulceration of fauces with greyish slough

**Diagnosis**
1. Heterophil antibodies (anti-sheep and horse RBC)
2. Lymphocytosis. Atypical lymphocytes in blood film
3. Anaemia absent (unlike leukaemia which blood picture can mimic)

CHICKENPOX
1. Cause — varicella zoster virus
2. Vesicular stomatitis and rash. Oral symptoms minor (but infection spreads from oral lesions)
3. Diagnosis can be confirmed by smear from vesicle showing similar features to those in herpetic stomatitis

*Note*: 1. Reactivation of virus (typically late in life) produces zoster
2. Both chickenpox and zoster infections can cause varicella in the non-immune

MEASLES
1. Koplik's spots — 'grains of salt' and bright erythema of buccal mucosa — specific early sign
2. Rash after a few days

*CANDIDA ALBICANS* INFECTIONS (CANDIDOSIS)

**Thrush**
1. Predominantly infants, immunosuppressed or debilitated patients
2. Invasion of epithelium by candidal hyphae
3. Epithelial proliferation and inflammatory infiltrate forming soft plaque
4. Creamy, scattered flecks or confluent plaque. Readily wiped off leaving red area
5. Angular stomatitis typically associated
6. Investigate possible underlying cause
7. Topical nystatin or amphotericin effective

**Diagnosis**
Gram stained smear — tangled masses of hyphae

**Angular stomatitis (cheilitis)**
1. Redness or ulceration at angle of mouth. Spread along skin folds (if present) at angle of mouth
2. Typical sign of leakage of candida-infected saliva from *any* type of intra-oral candidosis acute or chronic
3. Most often associated with denture stomatitis
4. Treatment — eradication of intra-oral infection with antifungal drugs

*Other causes of angular stomatitis*
1. Anaemia (possibly mediated by candidal infection)
2. *Staphylococcus aureus* and mixed staphylococcal and candidal infections

## Denture stomatitis
1. Proliferation of hyphae between denture and underlying mucosa. No tissue invasion
2. (i) Erythema of upper denture-bearing mucosa
   (ii) Usually no symptoms. Rarely sore ('denture sore mouth')
   (iii) Angular stomatitis often associated
3. Treatment — topical nystatin, amphotericin or miconazole
   Keep dentures in antiseptic (hypochlorite).

## Candidal leukoplakia and mucocutaneous candidosis syndromes
See White Lesions, page 80.

## SYPHILIS

### Primary
1. Ulcerating painless nodule on lip or tongue (may mimic carcinoma). Rare
2. Swollen, rubbery, discrete cervical nodes
3. Highly infective

### Diagnosis
History and smear (dark field examination). Many *T. pallidum* (difficult to differentiate from oral commensal spirochaetes). Serology negative

### Secondary
1. Mucous patches or snail track ulcers. Rare
2. Rash, typically symmetrical coppery macules
3. Generalised lymphadenopathy, fever and malaise

### Diagnosis
Serology and smears positive

### Tertiary
1. Gumma (*or* leukoplakia — see White Lesions, p. 80). Rare
2. Chronic inflammation and endarteritis. Central necrosis
3. Punched out ulcer, wash-leather floor, painless. Scarring and distortion (e.g. tongue) or perforation of palate
4. CNS or CVS syphilis often associated

### Diagnosis and management
1. Serology positive
2. Treatment (all stages) usually with penicillin

## GONOCOCCAL STOMATITIS
1. Probably from oro-genital contact. Rare
2. Acute widespread erythema and oedema with or without painful ulceration and exudate
3. Pharynx particularly, but any part of oral mucosa

4. Regional lymphadenopathy, fever and malaise, or asymptomatic
5. Smear — gram-negative diplococci in polymorphs
6. Culture swab to confirm
7. Treatment — penicillin, but resistant strains now prevalent

## TUBERCULOSIS
1. Complication of persistent pulmonary tuberculosis. Rare
2. Tuberculous granulomas with AFB and giant cells. Sometimes caseation. Destruction of epithelium and adjacent tissues
3. Typically, stellate ulcer with overhanging edges on dorsum of tongue. Pain in late stages

### Diagnosis and management
1. Biopsy. Ziehl-Neelsen stain for AFB (rarely positive in oral lesions)
2. Chest radiographs. Sputum culture
3. Systemic antibiotic treatment (e.g. isoniazid and rifampicin plus streptomycin or ethambutol)

## IMMUNOLOGICALLY MEDIATED OR OF DUBIOUS AETIOLOGY

### APHTHOUS STOMATITIS (RECURRENT APHTHAE)
1. Infiltration of epithelium by mononuclears, epithelial destruction and infiltration by polymorphs
2. Reported immunological findings
    (i) Serum antibodies to crude extracts of fetal oral mucosa
    (ii) Antibodies to bacterial *(Strep. sanguis)* antigens may cross-react with epithelial cells
    (iii) Cytotoxic activity of lymphocytes against oral epithelial cells
    (Clinical significance of *in vitro* immune phenomena uncertain and no reliable response to immunosuppressive treatment)
3. Folic acid, $B_{12}$ or iron deficiencies in 5 to 10 per cent
4. Family history frequently positive but genetic basis (if any) uncertain
5. Aphthae occasionally severe premenstrually or clear during pregnancy
6. Predominantly in non-smokers. Sometimes initiated by stopping smoking
7. Onset typically in childhood or adolescence. Often increasingly severe, peaking in early adult life
8. Temporary remissions common. Spontaneously self-limiting eventually
9. Non-masticatory mucosa affected. Types:
    (i) Minor aphthae. Ulcers 4 to 6 mm rounded shallow erythematous margin and sore. Common
    (ii) 'Herpetiform'. Many 2 to 3 mm ulcers. Widespread erythema. Uncommon
    (iii) Major aphthae. Ulcers typically 1 to 5 cm. May affect masticatory mucosa. Typically persist several months. Variable scarring. Uncommon

## Diagnosis and management
1. Biopsy — changes not specific but may be used to exclude other causes of ulceration
2. No useful serological tests
3. Diagnosis dependent on history and clinical features
4. Exclude B$_{12}$, folate or iron deficiency
5. Topical corticosteroids (e.g. hydrocortisone lozenges 2.5 mg tds) occasionally effective
6. Tetracycline mouth rinses 250 mg in water tds (effective in recent controlled trials)
7. Antiseptics (e.g. chlorhexidine) or zinc sulphate mouthwashes may help a little
8. Remedy any haematological deficiency — curative in folic acid deficiency especially

## BEHCET'S SYNDROME
1. Recurrent aphthae (minor or major), genital ulcers and uveitis
2. Many (but highly variable) systemic manifestations — thrombophlebitis, rashes, arthralgia, CNS involvement
3. Wide variation in incidence in different countries — particularly common in Turkey and Japan
4. Immunological basis speculative and treatment empirical. No reliable response to immunosuppressive treatment
5. No absolute criteria of diagnosis. No immunological tests of value. Recurrent oral and genital ulcers the most constant feature

## LICHEN PLANUS
1. Common. Especially middle-aged women
2. Cause unknown. Occasionally drug-associated (p. 78). History of emotional stress common
3. Pathology
   (i) White lesions. Hyperkeratosis. Saw-tooth profile of rete ridges, liquefaction degeneration of basal cells, dense subepithelial band of lymphocytes (mainly T cells)
   (ii) Atrophic lesions. Thinning and flattening of epithelium, similar inflammatory infiltrate
   (iii) Erosions. Destruction of epithelium with fibrinous superficial exudate. Widespread inflammation
4. Lacy pattern of well-defined white striae typically symmetrically on buccal mucosae. Painful, atrophic (red) areas or erosions (ulcers) often associated
5. Dorsum of tongue often, lips or palate rarely affected. Gingival lesions usually atrophic ('desquamative gingivitis')
6. Dermal lesions (violaceous papules with microscopic striae on surface) occasionally associated. Typically flexor surfaces of limbs
7. Good response to potent topical corticosteroids (e.g. betamethasone valerate). Systemic corticosteroids occasionally needed

**Diagnosis**
1. Appearance and distribution of lesions often distinctive
2. Biopsy necessary in atypical cases
3. Differential diagnosis from lupus erythematosus, see p. 121.
4. Occasionally progresses to dysplasia or malignant change but premalignant potential controversial

## PEMPHIGUS VULGARIS
1. Intra-epithelial vesicles. Separation of epithelial cells due to loss of interepithelial attachment (acantholysis). Ulceration
2. Circulating auto-antibodies against epithelial intercellular substance. Immunoglobulin and complement localised along intercellular boundaries by immunofluorescence (frozen section)
3. Patients usually middle-aged. Mainly women
4. Fragile vesicles and ulcers in mouth. Frequently precede skin lesions
5. Widespread vesicles and ulcers of skin. Fatal if untreated

**Diagnosis and management**
1. Acantholytic cells in smears from vesicle fluid. Confirm by biopsy and immunofluorescence microscopy (see above)
2. Immunosuppressive treatment (corticosteroids plus azathioprine) life-saving
3. Other auto-immune disease sometimes associated

## MUCOUS MEMBRANE PEMPHIGOID
1. Loss of attachment of epithelium to connective tissue producing subepithelial vesicles
2. Complement and sometimes immunoglobulin localised at basement membrane level in about 80 per cent, by immunofluorescence
3. Onset typically in late middle age
4. Vesicles often persist on oral mucosa. Rupture leaves chronic painful ulcers. Gingivae may be main site ('desquamative gingivitis')
5. Very indolent. Other mucous membranes, especially eyes, may be affected leading to scarring. Sight may be damaged
6. Skin lesions uncommon and minor

**Diagnosis**
1. Biopsy and immunofluorescence microscopy (see above)
2. Rarely circulating auto-antibodies
3. Topical corticosteroids often effective for oral lesions. Systemic steroids needed if eyes or other mucous membranes affected

## BULLOUS ERYTHEMA MULTIFORME (STEVENS-JOHNSON SYNDROME)

1. Occasionally post-infective (mycoplasmal or herpetic) or drug-associated (e.g. sulphonamides). More often no cause identifiable
2. Intra-epithelial vesiculation, ulceration and inflammation. Biopsy may be diagnostic
3. Clinically, mainly young adults. May recur
4. Mouth most common (often the only) site. Bleeding, swelling and crusting of lips, widespread ill-defined ulceration of oral mucosa due to rupture of vesicles
5. Rash (target lesions or erythema) — involvement of other mucous membranes (especially eyes and genitalia). Fever and malaise sometimes. Usually self-limiting
6. No specific treatment. Systemic corticosteroids may help

## LUPUS ERYTHEMATOSUS
See page 121

## MUCOSAL REACTIONS TO DRUGS

### LOCAL
1. Chemical irritation (chromic acid, phenol, unswallowed tablets, e.g. aspirin, edrophonium, etc.)
2. Disturbance of oral flora (candidosis due to topical antibiotics, especially tetracycline)

### SYSTEMICALLY MEDIATED
1. Depression of marrow
    (i) Agranulocytosis (chloramphenicol, sulphamethoxazole, phenylbutazone, antithyroid agents)
   (ii) Purpura (apronal, chloramphenicol)
  (iii) Folate deficiency (phenytoin)
2. Depression of cell-mediated immunity. Immunosuppressive treatment (fungal and viral infections of mucosa)
3. Lichenoid reactions (gold, antimalarials, non-steroidal anti-inflammatory drugs methyldopa)
4. Bullous erythema multiforme (long-acting sulphonamides, phenobarbitone(?))
5. Ulceration by cytotoxic drugs, especially methotrexate
6. Exfoliative dermatitis and stomatitis (gold, phenylbutazone, barbiturates)

*Other effects*
1. Gingival hyperplasia (phenytoin, cyclosporin)
2. Pigmentation (heavy metals, phenothiazines)
3. Dry mouth (p. 98)

## CHRONIC KERATOSES (LEUKOPLAKIAS, WHITE LESIONS)

### Significance
1. Increased risk of malignant change *but*
2. Few white lesions premalignant (3 to 5 per cent after 10 years)
3. Biopsy essential
4. Epithelial dysplasia — only available index of malignant potential but prognosis uncertain

### General microscopic features
1. Hyperortho- or parakeratosis
2. Prominent granular cell layer if orthokeratotic
3. Prickle cell layer may be hyperplastic (acanthosis) or atrophic
4. Inflammatory infiltrate in corium often associated but variable in character and distribution
5. Dysplasia of epithelium sometimes present (see p. 82)

### WHITE SPONGE NAEVUS
1. Autosomal dominant
2. Epithelial hyperplasia. Thick, oedematous ('basket-weave') superficial plaque. No inflammation
3. Irregular white soft thickening, typically of whole oral mucosa
4. Fragments detach or chewed off
5. Anal or other mucosa may be affected
6. No treatment. Reassure

### FRICTIONAL KERATOSIS
1. Hyperkeratosis, acanthosis (usually). Varying chronic inflammatory infiltrate
2. Clinically, chronic white thickening related to source of chronic low-grade trauma
3. Resolves rapidly with removal of irritant (diagnostic) — if not, biopsy

### SMOKER'S KERATOSIS
1. Typically pipe-smokers after many years
2. Hyperkeratosis, variable inflammatory infiltrate. Inflammation of palatal glands
3. Keratosis of palatal mucosa. Mucous glands swollen with red orifices. Area under denture unaffected
4. Rapid regression if smoking stopped
5. Possible risk of cancer. Usually *not* in area of keratosis (e.g. usually below and lingual to $\overline{8}$)

## SYPHILITIC LEUKOPLAKIA
1. Occasional feature of tertiary syphilis. Now exceedingly rare
2. Hyperkeratosis, variable irregular acanthosis sometimes with dysplasia. Chronic inflammation, plasma cells and endarteritis deeply
3. Tough irregular whitish plaque. Dorsum of tongue
4. Risk of malignant change high
5. Biopsy and serological examination
6. No response to antisyphilitic treatment (penicillin should be given for systemic lesions)
7. CVS or CNS disease often associated

## CHRONIC CANDIDOSIS
1. Invasion of epithelium by hyphae (stain with PAS). Parakeratosis, inflammatory exudate in plaque. Acanthosis and chronic inflammation
2. 'Idiopathic' or rare mucocutaneous candidosis syndrome
3. Tongue, buccal commisures or, less often, other sites. Tough, adherent, whitish plaque of variable thickness. Sometimes speckled
4. Chronic angular stomatitis may be associated

**Diagnosis**
1. Smear (gram stain) and biopsy (PAS stain) essential. Dysplasia sometimes present
2. Investigation for endocrinopathy (e.g. hypoparathyroidism) may be indicated
3. Cell-mediated immunity occasionally impaired
4. Imidazole antifungals (e.g. miconazole) probably most effective
5. Possibly increased risk of malignant change

## CHRONIC MUCOCUTANEOUS CANDIDOSIS SYNDROMES

*Typical features*
1. Rare
2. Most start in infancy as persistent thrush. Chronic (leukoplakia-like) lesions develop in childhood
3. Severe types frequently with defect of cell-mediated immunity (CMI)
4. Mouth often predominantly or solely affected

*Types*
1. Familial (autosomal recessive).
   Persistent oral candidal 'leukoplakia' main feature
2. Candida-endocrinopathy syndrome (autosomal recessive).
   Hypoparathyroidism, Addison's disease or other auto-immune disease associated
3. Diffuse (candida 'granuloma').
   Severe oral candidosis, proliferative skin lesions, bacterial infections, defective CMI often
4. Late onset, thymoma syndrome.
   Late middle age, thymoma, myasthenia gravis, anaemia, defective CMI, candidosis or other infections

## LICHEN PLANUS
1. Lesions occasionally plaque-like, especially on dorsum of tongue
2. Other features of lichen planus, if present, assist diagnosis
3. Biopsy

## IDIOPATHIC KERATOSES
1. No cause detectable in majority of leukoplakias
2. Women of middle age or over, probably mainly affected
3. Variable appearance. Thick widespread plaques to minimal thin, whitish areas, sometimes with erythema
4. Pathology highly variable — from severe hyperkeratosis and hyperplasia to minimal parakeratosis with or without dysplasia
5. Sublingual butterfly lesions — symmetrical, wrinkled surface, sharply-defined irregular outline. No peripheral erythema. Typically, under-surface of anterior tongue and adjacent floor of mouth. High risk of carcinoma
6. Biopsy essential. Repeat as necessary if dysplastic or change in clinical character
7. Prognosis unpredictable. Risk of malignant change probably high in this group
8. Management. Keep under observation if dysplasia absent. If dysplasia develops, manage as below

## SUBLINGUAL KERATOSIS*
1. Typically soft, butterfly-like white lesion with wrinkled surface on underside of anterior tongue and adjacent floor of mouth but variable appearances
2. Women slightly more commonly affected
3. Malignant change in 10 to 25 per cent reported

**Diagnosis**
Biopsy essential for detection of dysplasia or malignant change

*Formerly classified as an epithelial naevus

## DYSPLASTIC (DYSKERATOTIC) LEUKOPLAKIA

1. Diagnosis only by histology
2. Features of epithelial dysplasia (atypia, dyskeratosis). Varying combinations of:
   (i) Nuclear hyperchromatism
   (ii) Increased nuclear-cytoplasmic ratio
   (iii) Nuclear pleomorphism
   (vi) Deep cell keratinisation
   (v) Loss of polarity
   (vi) Disorganisation of progress of maturation
   (vii) Increased (sometimes abnormal) mitoses
   (viii) Epithelium often thin (atrophic)
3. *Carcinoma-in-situ.* Severe dysplasia with abnormalities throughout epithelium (top-to-bottom change) but no invasion
4. No characteristic clinical appearance. May be white, red and velvety (erythroplasia) or speckled
5. Speckled leukoplakias (white flecks or nodules on atrophic, erythematous base) and, especially, erythroplasias most susceptible to malignant change
6. Prognosis unpredictable. Carcinomatous change often within 6 months to 2 years. Some remain static or, rarely, regress
7. Management unsatisfactory. Wide excision and grafting possibly effective but no proven value. Keep under 3-monthly observation. Repeat biopsy if lesion changes in any way. Treat carcinoma, if it develops, immediately by accepted means

*Note*: Most carcinomas probably do not pass through clinically detectable premalignant stage. Dysplastic lesions much less common than overt carcinomas

## EARLY CARCINOMA

1. Well-differentiated carcinomas may produce surface keratin. Transiently indistinguishable clinically from small benign white lesions
2. No symptoms, but rapid progress to typical carcinoma
3. Biopsy all small white lesions and erythroplasias without overt cause, especially in older patients

## SKIN GRAFTS

1. Regular shape, sharply-defined margin, smooth surface. Hairs sometimes present
2. History diagnostic but original pathology (e.g. carcinoma or candidosis) can recur in graft

## SUMMARY OF IMPORTANT CAUSES OF ORAL ULCERATION

1. Traumatic
   (i) Mechanical irritation
   (ii) Radiation mucositis
2. Chemical
   (i) Drug reactions (local)
   (ii) Drug reactions (systemically mediated)
3. Infective
   (i) Herpetic stomatitis
   (ii) Herpes zoster
   (iii) Hand, foot and mouth disease
   (iv) Herpangina
   (v) Acute ulcerative gingivitis
   (vi) Tuberculosis
   (vii) Syphilis
4. Neoplastic
   Carcinoma and other tumours
5. Immunologically mediated or dubious aetiology
   (i) Aphthous stomatitis
   (ii) Erosive lichen planus
   (iii) Pemphigus vulgaris
   (iv) Mucous membrane pemphigoid
   (v) Acute erythema multiforme

## LESIONS OF THE TONGUE

1. Sore tongue
2. Geographical tongue
3. Median rhomboid glossitis
4. Hairy tongue

### SORE TONGUE

1. Stomatitis (any) or other types of ulcer (e.g. carcinoma)
2. Anaemia
3. Nutritional (very rare)
4. Psychogenic (usually depression — common)

### Anaemia

*Causes*
1. Iron deficiency
2. Pernicious anaemia
3. Folate deficiency

*Signs on tongue*
1. General depapillation and redness or
2. Patchy red areas or
3. Normal papillation and colour

**Diagnosis**
1. Medical history, e.g. heavy menstrual losses, peptic ulcer, etc.
2. Laboratory investigation: Hb., MCV, etc.; direct film; serum B12, folate, etc. as appropriate

   (*Note*: Hb may still be within normal limits)

### *Nutritional*

$B_2$ (riboflavin) or $B_6$ (nicotinic acid) deficiency — very rarely confirmed

## GEOGRAPHICAL TONGUE
1. ? Developmental. Family history relatively common
2. Central area of loss of filiform papillae, mild superficial inflammation. Polymorph infiltration of surface epithelium at margins
3. Irregular smooth red areas, often with white margin, on dorsum of tongue. Pattern varies from week to week
4. Sometimes sore

## MEDIAN RHOMBOID GLOSSITIS
1. ? Developmental. Some cases show chronic candidosis histologically
2. Site: dorsum of tongue, midline, just anterior to circumvalate papillae
3. Appearances:
   a. rhomboid or ovoid
   b. smooth and red *or* white, *or*
   c. lobulated

## HAIRY OR BLACK TONGUE
1. Variable overgrowth of filiform papillae and bacterial proliferation
2. Pigmentation due to chromogenic bacteria or fungi
3. Hairiness and pigmentation variably associated
4. Topical tetracycline can cause overgrowth of chromogenic bacteria. Causes rarely otherwise found

# Tumours and tumour-like swellings of soft tissues

1. Hyperplastic lesions
    (i) Polyps, epulides and granulomas
    (ii) Pyogenic granuloma and pregnancy epulis
    (iii) Papillary hyperplasia of palate
    (iv) Giant cells epulis
2. Epithelial tumours — benign
    (i) Squamous cell papilloma
    (ii) Adenoma
3. Epithelial tumours — malignant
    (i) Squamous cell carcinoma
    (ii) Adenocarcinomas
4. Connective tissue tumours — benign
    (i) Neurofibroma
    (ii) Lipoma
    (iii) Haemangiomas
    (iv) Lymphangioma
    (v) Others
5. Connective tissue tumours — malignant
    (i) Fibrosarcoma and neurofibrosarcoma
    (ii) Rhabdomyosarcoma
6. Pigmented naevi and malignant melanomas
7. Lymphomas and plasmacytoma
8. Miscellaneous non-neoplastic lesions
    (i) Granular cell myoblastoma
    (ii) Granular cell epulis of the newborn

*Note:* (1) Histopathology of many soft tissue tumours essentially same as counterparts in jaws (p. 53) (2) All specimens should be examined histologically to confirm diagnosis

## HYPERPLASTIC LESIONS

### FIBROUS POLYPS, EPULIDES AND GRANULOMAS
1. Most common oral soft tissue 'tumours'
2. Chronic irritation, infection, inflammation, proliferation of granulation tissue, progressive fibrosis and epithelialisation
3. Typical sites. Gum margin (fibrous epulis) denture margin (denture granuloma), cheek (fibrous polyp)
4. Excise adequately. Remove any source of irritation
5. Confirm by microscopy

*Note*: 'Epulis' refers only to *site* of lesion
Epulides may be:
1. Fibrous (most cases)
2. Pregnancy 'tumours'
3. Giant cell (occasionally)
4. Malignant (particularly secondary carcinoma) — rarely Biopsy therefore essential

### PYOGENIC GRANULOMA
1. Highly vascular, exuberant granulation tissue, with often intense inflammatory cellular infiltrate
2. Responds to excision

### PREGNANCY EPULIS
1. May be indistinguishable from and regarded by some as merely a pyogenic granuloma
2. Typically associated with pregnancy gingivitis
3. Occasionally lacks inflammatory infiltrate and consists of thin-walled vascular spaces with proliferation of endothelium in loose, delicate, oedematous connective tissue
4. May resolve post-partum if oral hygiene good

### PAPILLARY HYPERPLASIA OF PALATE
1. Multiple small nodules of hyperplastic epithelium and connective tissue — variable inflammation superimposed
2. Nodular area in vault of hard palate. May be aggravated by infection under denture
3. Relieve infection or other irritant if inflamed

GIANT CELL EPULIS
1. Multinucleate giant cells in vascular stroma of plump spindle cells covered by epithelium
2. Aetiology unknown — non-neoplastic
3. Clinically, typically red, haemorrhagic and soft
4. Usually anterior to molars before age 30. More common in females
5. Slight superficial bone erosion sometimes
6. Excision usually curative

*Note*: Endosteal giant cell granuloma may erode through bone producing broad-based, dome-shaped or flattened protrusion with extensive area of radiolucency in jaw

## EPITHELIAL TUMOURS

SQUAMOUS CELL PAPILLOMA
1. Branched finger-like processes of stratified squamous epithelium with vascular core. Variable keratinisation
2. Warty (papillated) swelling. White (if keratinised) or pink. Pedunculated or sessile
3. Excise

### Adenomas
1. Origin from minor salivary glands (p. 99)
2. Most often on posterior palate or cheek. Slightly lobulated, rubbery swelling mobile on deeper tissues. Slow-growing. Often traumatic ulceration of surface
3. Adequate excision curative

### SQUAMOUS CELL CARCINOMA (INTRA-ORAL)
Most common and important oral malignant tumour

### Aetiology
1. Unknown in most cases
2. Epidemiological association with pipe-smoking
3. Strong association with tobacco use in India
4. In US epidemiological association with cirrhosis (usually alcoholic) of liver reported
5. Increased cigarette and alcohol consumption associated with *declining* oral cancer incidence in Britain, i.e. no aetiological relationship here
6. Carcinoma in syphilitic leukoplakia exceedingly rare now

## Histopathology

1. Epithelial hyperplasia, invasion and destruction of surrounding tissue
2. Variable degrees of epithelial dysplasia (p. 82) and loss of differentiation
3. Deep keratinisation and formation of cell nests and/or surface keratinisation in well-differentiated tumours
4. Typically, dense inflammatory, mainly lymphocytic, infiltrate around growing edges
5. Necrosis and ulceration with infection in later stages
6. Well-differentiated squamous cell carcinoma in over 90 per cent. Deep invasion and spread to regional lymph nodes

## Clinical aspects

1. Age: 98 per cent over 40
2. Sex: Male to female ratio approx.2:1.(Generally declining in males. Equal sex ratio in SE England)
3. Majority of tumours in horse-shoe shaped area of edges of tongue, adjacent floor of mouth, lingual alveolar margin to oropharynx
4. Tongue, most common intra-oral site (dorsum of tongue exceedingly rarely affected in absence of syphilis). Vault of palate hardly ever affected

## Clinical stages

1. Early:Small (5 to 6 mm) nodule, white or red patch or erosion; few or no symptoms
2. Middle:usually ulcer with hard raised edges and granulating floor. Rarely, cauliflower (exophytic) mass. Increasing fixation. Often pain or tenderness. Lymph nodes may be involved
3. Late:extensive destruction, fixation, difficulty in eating, talking or swallowing. Pain typically severe. Lymph nodes involved

## Treatment

Early — excision or radiotherapy
Later — radiotherapy with or without surgery. (Overall about 80 per cent irradiated)

## Prognosis

5-year survival rates for tongue (all stages) 37 to 45 per cent

## CANCER OF THE LIP
1. More common than any single intra-oral site
2. Main aetiological factor — exposure to sunshine, especially if fair-skinned. Geographical distribution accordingly
3. Rare in women
4. Well-differentiated squamous cell carcinoma
5. Early lesion — small (5 mm), persistent, crusted patch on lower lip.
   Progress to typical malignant ulcer and spread to nodes if neglected
6. Diagnosis preferably by excision biopsy of small lesion
7. Treatment; surgery or radiotherapy
8. 5-year survival rate 80 to 90 per cent

## VERRUCOUS CARCINOMA
1. Uncommon variant
2. Histopathology. Extensive papilloma-like proliferation, hyperkeratosis, defined lower border to epithelial downgrowths, dysplasia minimal or absent, 'benign' appearance. Dysplasia and invasion develop late
3. Typically in elderly patients
4. Widespread white, warty or craggy mass
5. Slow progress. Spread to lymph nodes late
6. Good prognosis if widely excised. (Irradiation may induce anaplastic change with poor prognosis)

## PREMALIGNANT LESIONS
1. Epithelial dysplasia, for microscopic features, see page 82)
2. Clinical appearances
   (i) Red patch (erythroplasia)
   (ii) Erosion
   (iii) White patch, or
   (iv) Speckled red and white patch
   Note: no specific appearance
3. Premalignant nature of lesion proved only by progress to cancer. Dysplastic lesions occasionally regress or remain stationary

## ADENOCARCINOMAS
Uncommon oral cancers of minor salivary glands (p. 99)

## METASTATIC CARCINOMA
1. Carcinomas from distant site (e.g. gut or bronchus) may mimic benign epulis. Confirm by biopsy
2. Rare

## BENIGN CONNECTIVE TISSUE TUMOURS
Examples:
1. *Neurofibroma*. Rarely associated with neurofibromatosis. Usually neurilemoma. Typically elongated spindle cells with palisaded nuclei. Firm smooth swelling. Excise
2. *Lipoma*. Fat cells with fibrous capsule. Soft, yellowish swelling usually of buccal mucosa. Excise
3. *Haemangioma*. Usually a hamartoma
    (i) Capillary or cavernous
    (ii) Localised, prominent, purplish, blood-filled compressible swelling or widespread red area
    (iii) May be associated with facial naevus
    (iv) Avoid treatment unless frequent or profuse bleeding
    (v) Cryosurgery useful
4. *Lymphangioma*
    (i) Small or dilated vessels filled with lymph
    (ii) Typically almost colourless
    (iii) May 'go black' (bleeding into lymphatic spaces)
    (iv) Rarely extensive, causing macroglossia or generalised enlargement of other tissue
    (v) Excise if troublesome and feasible

## SARCOMAS
1. All uncommon — main types, see below
2. No specific clinical features. Typically soft, often rapidly growing swellings in younger patients
3. Diagnosis by biopsy
4. Treatment. Surgery, radiotherapy and/or chemotherapy according to type. Prognosis variable, often poor

## FIBROSARCOMA
1. Occasionally post-irradiation
2. Bundles of fibroblasts, variable pleomorphism, mitoses and collagen production according to differentiation
3. Progressive, invasive
4. Metastases uncommon, especially if well-differentiated
5. Excise radically

## RHABDOMYOSARCOMA
1. Histopathology variable — examples of features:
    (i) Pleomorphic type. Large, racquet-, tadpole-, strap- or ribbon-shaped cells. Cross-striation sometimes seen
    (ii) Alveolar. Small dark cells hanging from walls of fusiform spaces or free in interior. Connective tissue stroma
2. Rapid growth and spread — mainly by blood stream

## KAPOSI'S SARCOMA
1. Seen virtually only in immunosuppressed and Acquired Immune Deficiency syndrome (p. 125) patients in the Western world
2. Clinically consists of fleshy, purplish soft nodules affecting palate, lip or tongue particularly
3. May be solitary or part of widespread disease
4. Histologically resembles rapidly proliferating granulation tissue, with endothelial and spindle cell proliferation and many vascular spaces. Areas of haemorrhage and haemosiderin deposition.
5. Originates in endothelial cells

## PIGMENTED NAEVI
1. Naevus cells in subepithelial connective tissue. Variable melanin production
2. Junctional activity (melanocytes in and 'dropping off' basal layer of epithelium) may be associated but usually benign in children
3. Circumscribed brown to black area of mucosa. Non-progressive
4. Excise for biopsy

## MALIGNANT MELANOMA
1. Malignant melanocytes in clear areas in epithelium and spreading down into connective tissue (junctional activity and invasion). Tumour cells pleomorphic, round or spindle-shaped. Variable melanin production and inflammatory reaction. Biopsy essential
2. Types:
   (i) Superficial spreading
   (ii) Nodular invasive. Prognosis related to depth of invasion
3. Red to black in colour. Flat area of pigmentation or well-defined nodule
4. Spread to regional lymph nodes and blood stream
5. Excise widely. Prognosis poor except for limited superficial lesions

## LYMPHOMAS AND RELATED TUMOURS
1. Any type of lymphoma may affect oral tissues
   All rare. Cervical lymph nodes more frequently the early site (p. 102)
2. Typically rapidly growing destructive, soft swellings, often ulcerating (trauma)
3. Diagnosis by biopsy
4. Oral lesions may be primary (then disseminate) or secondary
5. Prognosis poor (except solitary plasmacytoma — (see p. 59)

## MISCELLANEOUS TUMOUR-LIKE LESIONS

### GRANULAR CELL TUMOUR ('MYOBLASTOMA')
1. Probably derived from Schwann cells
2. Enlarged cells with abundant granular cytoplasm and small nuclei. Granular cells intermingle with or replace muscle fibres
3. Pseudo-epitheliomatous hyperplasia of overlying epithelium may closely mimic carcinoma
4. Tongue, most common site. Typically, painless firm swelling
5. Excise — recurrence rare

### GRANULAR CELL TUMOUR (EPULIS) OF NEWBORN
1. Rare
2. Pedunculated or sessile swelling usually on upper alveolar ridge
3. Structure — as above but lacks pseudo-epitheliomatous hyperplasia.

# Salivary gland disease

**Chief complaints**
1. Pain and/or
2. Swelling and/or
3. Dry mouth

*Note:* Hypersecretion not an entity. Sialorrhea (dribbling) due to poor neuromuscular control (typically in Parkinson's disease), dysphagia, mental defect or neurotic complaint

SALIVARY GLAND PAIN
1. Stones or other causes of obstruction
2. Mumps
3. Salivary gland cancer

*Rare causes*
1. Sjögren's syndrome
2. Acute ascending parotitis
3. Recurrent parotitis

SALIVARY GLAND SWELLING
1. Mumps
2. Tumours
3. Sjögren's syndrome
4. Drug-induced
5. Ascending parotitis

*Rare causes*
1. Mikulicz disease (lymphoepithelial lesion) and syndrome
2. Sarcoidosis
3. Actinomycosis (p. 93)
4. Sialosis

DRY MOUTH
1. Organic disease of glands
   (i) Sjögren's syndrome
   (ii) Irradiation damage
   (iii) Mumps and other infections (temporary)
2. Functional causes
   (i) Drugs with anticholinergic or sympathomimetic effects
   (p. 98)
   (ii) Chronic anxiety states
   (iii) Dehydration (e.g. diarrhoea and vomiting, severe
   haemorrhage)

## STONES, OBSTRUCTION AND CYSTS

### Duct obstruction

*Causes*
1. Calculi
2. Stenosis (secondary to stones, infection, surgery or tumour)
3. Papillary obstruction. (Usually due to local trauma and
   inflammation)  eg: DENTURE CLASPS , CYSTS

## CALCULI

### Clinical features may be
1. Pain related to eating
2. Pain and swelling (infection secondary to duct obstruction)
3. Local pain and swelling due to infection and inflammation round
   stone near orifice
4. Palpable stone (near orifice of duct)
5. No symptoms, but stones seen in radiograph

### Diagnosis
1. Calculus palpable or visible
2. Radiographs (calcified stones — about 20 per cent of
   submandibular and 40 per cent of parotid stones nonopaque. 25
   per cent of salivary calculi are multiple)

### Management
1. Radiographs and sialogram for site and cause of obstruction and,
   possibly, other pathology
2. Remove stone or repair stricture
3. Excise gland if damage severe or infection recurrent
4. Antibiotics if acute infection associated

## SIALADENITIS

### MUMPS
1. Viral infection. Mainly children
2. Prodromal fever, malaise, sore throat
3. Acute, painful tender parotid swelling. Usually bilateral
4. Groove behind ramus filled in. Tip of earlobe everted
5. Overlying skin normal
6. Orifice of duct inflamed
7. Submandibular or sublingual glands occasionally also involved

#### Diagnosis
1. History (acute parotid swelling with mild, febrile illness — no history of mumps earlier in life — known contact with other cases)
2. Serology , rising titre of complement-fixing antibodies (rarely needed)

#### Management
Analgesics and bed rest. Refer to family doctor

### SUPPURATIVE PAROTITIS
1. Complication of dry mouth (especially in Sjögren's syndrome debilitated patients or post-operative)
2. Typically staphylococcal, sometimes pneumococcal
3. Pain and swelling. Warm red, shiny overlying skin
4. Regional lymphadenopathy
5. Fever and malaise
6. Pus from duct orifice
7. Xerostomia

#### Diagnosis and management
1. Pus (milk parotid duct if necessary) for smears, culture and sensitivity
2. Appropriate antibiotic in high dose. Restore hydration

### CHRONIC SIALADENITIS
1. Usually complication of chronic duct obstruction
2. Intermittent, painful swelling of gland
3. Duct orifice often red; sometimes purulent or salty discharge

#### Management
1. Remove any obstruction, or
2. Excise gland if necessary

RECURRENT PAROTITIS
1. Cause unknown — probably infective
2. Adults or children
3. Sudden onset of pain and swelling. Beads of pus from duct
4. Attacks up to a week duration
5. Usually self-limiting ultimately

## SJÖGREN'S AND SICCA SYNDROMES

1. Definitions
    (i) Sjögren's syndrome — dry mouth, dry eyes and rheumatoid arthritis or other connective tissue disease
    (ii) Sicca syndrome — dry mouth and dry eyes *without* associated connective tissue disease
        Sjögren's and sicca syndromes have in common their effects on gland function and histopathology but also differ in the immunological abnormalities. Sicca syndrome also tends to have more severe effects on the glands
2. Infiltration of gland by lymphocytes. Destruction of acini but some proliferation of duct epithelium (epimyoepithelial islands)
3. Common; about 15 per cent of patients with rheumatoid arthritis and 30 per cent of patients with systemic lupus erythematosus
4. Mainly women over middle age
5. Parotid swelling in minority
6. Pain unusual

### Oral features
1. Xerostomia
2. Pebbly lobulation of dorsum of tongue
3. Severe periodontal disease or dental caries
4. Candidal infection — sore mouth and angular stomatitis

### Ocular changes
Early keratoconjunctivitis sicca asymptomatic. Later 'gritty' eyes; conjunctivitis and progressive damange

### Diagnosis
1. Exclude other causes, especially drugs
2. Parotid flow rate after stimulation (normal 1 to 1.5ml/min, reduced to approx. 0.4 to 0.25)
3. Labial gland biopsy (good correlation with parotid changes)
4. Sialography. Snow-storm pattern ('sialectasis')
5. Ophthalmological investigation. Essential in *all* patients even if no symptoms

*Serology*
1. Rheumatoid factor in 40 to 90 per cent
2. Anti-nuclear factor in 40 to 90 per cent
3. Anti-salivary duct antibody in 10 to 60 per cent

*Note:* Figures differ in full-blown Sjögren's and sicca syndromes

## Management
1. Give artificial saliva. (Methylcellulose solution or glycerin and lemon)
2. Deal with any caries, periodontal disease or candidosis
3. Watch for ocular changes. Repeat eye investigations as necessary

## Complications
1. Damage to sight
2. Caries, periodontal disease or candidosis
3. Ascending parotitis
4. Lymphoma. Late, uncommon but higher risk in sicca syndrome

## MIKULICZ DISEASE (BENIGN LYMPHOEPITHELIAL LESION)
1. Histologically the same as Sjögren's syndrome
2. Functional effects or serological abnormalities not detectable
3. Probably not a distinct entity

## MIKULICZ SYNDROME
1. Salivary and lacrimal swelling due to definable disease, e.g. lymphoma or sarcoidosis
2. Clinically, swelling may be severe and widespread ('hamster' appearance)

## SIALOSIS
Painless multiglandular hypertrophy of serous cells and fatty replacement — rare

## RADIATION DAMAGE
1. Common complication of irradiation of head and neck region
2. Destruction and fibrous replacement of secretory tissue. Persistent xerostomia
3. Caries and periodontal disease typically severe
4. Redness and soreness of mucosa (after healing of radiation mucositis) and angular stomatitis due to candidosis

**Management**
1. As for Sjögren's. Caries prevention (fluorides and no sweets), restorative treatment and meticulous oral hygiene
2. Avoid extractions. High risk of radiation-associated osteomyelitis (p. 45)

## DRUG-INDUCED XEROSTOMIA

**Drugs with anticholinergic effects**
1. Atropine and analogues (e.g. ipratropium)
2. Tricyclic antidepressants
3. Antihistamines
4. Antiemetics
5. Major (phenothiazine) tranquillisers
6. Some antihypertensives (especially ganglion-blockers)

**Drugs with sympathomimetic actions**
1. 'Cold cures' containing ephedrine, etc.
2. Decongestants
3. Bronchodilators
4. Appetite suppressants
5. Amphetamines

## DRUG-ASSOCIATED SALIVARY SWELLING

1. Uncommon
2. Possible causes — phenylbutazone, iodine compounds, thiouracil, catecholamines, sulphonamides, chlorhexidine

## SALIVARY GLAND TUMOURS

73 per cent in parotids, 5 to 10 per cent of tumours in intraoral glands. About 70 per cent are pleomorphic adenomas

INTRAORAL SALIVARY GLAND TUMOURS
1. Main sites — posterior palate and cheek
2. Benign tumours (usually pleomorphic adenoma), slow growing
3. No pain or tenderness. Mucosa normal unless traumatised
4. Firm, rubbery, lobulated often with bluish tinge
5. Malignant tumours often not distinguishable in early stages
6. Higher proportion of intraoral tumours malignant than in parotids

**Features of malignant tumours**
1. Rapid growth
2. Pain
3. Hard texture
4. Ulceration
5. Spread to regional lymph nodes

**Diagnosis**
Confirmation of diagnosis by histopathology

PAROTID TUMOURS
1. Firm swelling obliterating groove behind ramus
2. Features indicative of malignancy as above. Also facial palsy

**Pathology**
1. Benign
    (i) Pleomorphic adenoma
    (ii) Monomorphic adenoma
2. Intermediate
    (i) Muco-epidermoid tumour. (Occasional malignant variants)
    (ii) Acinic cell tumour. (Occasional malignant variants)
3. Malignant
   Epithelial
    (i) Adenoid cystic carcinoma
    (ii) Adenocarcinoma
    (iii) Squamous cell carcinoma
    (iv) Malignant change in pleomorphic adenoma
4. Non-epithelial
   Lymphomas

PLEOMORPHIC ADENOMA
Mixed pattern. Typically:
1. Duct-like structures
2. Myxomatous or cartilage-like tissue
3. Sheets of darkly-staining cells
4. Foci of squamous metaplasia
5. Fibrous capsule with compressed acini at periphery
6. Responds to adequate excision

MUCOEPIDERMOID TUMOUR
1. Mucous cells, often producing microcysts
2. Areas of epidermoid (squamous) cells
3. Usually responds to wide excision. Variable degrees of
   malignancy possible

ADENOID CYSTIC CARCINOMA
1. Swiss cheese (cribriform) pattern of small, darkly-staining
   uniform cells
2. Widely infiltrative and perineural spread
3. Excision plus irradiation sometimes effective

## CARCINOMAS

1. Adeno-and squamous cell carcinomas essentially similar structure to those in other sites
2. Malignant change in pleomorphic adenoma
    (i) Rare
    (ii) Typically long history then acceleration of growth and/or pain
    (iii) Histologically, area of carcinoma within pleomorphic adenoma
    (iv) Typically adenocarcinoma but variable appearances

## NECROTISING SIALOMETAPLASIA

1. Necrosis of gland lobules. Multiple islands of squamous epithelium in fibrous stroma with inflammatory infiltrate (rare in UK)
2. Tumour-like palatal mass often ulcerated
3. Typically adult males
4. Biopsy confirmatory
5. May heal spontaneously after 1 or 2 months
   Otherwise excise

## CYSTS OF SALIVARY GLANDS

### RANULA

1. Retention cyst of floor of mouth
2. Superficial, soft, fluctuant and bluish
3. Usually unilateral, 2 or 3 cm in diameter
   Occasionally large and bilateral
4. Histopathology. Thin fibrous wall with flattened ductal (cuboidal) epithelial lining
5. Excise cyst and gland

### MUCOUS EXTRAVASATION CYST (MUCOCOELE)

1. Commonest cyst of oral soft tissues
2. Minor salivary glands (particularly lip), affected
3. Pathogenesis. Injury to duct, escape and pooling of saliva in superficial connective tissue and inflammation. Coalescence of pools of saliva forms cyst with connective tissue wall
4. Rarely, duct obstruction produces retention cyst with epithelial lining
5. Clinically, superficial swelling typically 1 cm in diameter, hemispherical, fluctuant, bluish
6. Excise cyst and underlying minor gland
7. Biopsy

# Swellings in the neck

## CAUSES

SWELLINGS OF CERVICAL LYMPH NODES
1. Lymphadenitis (dental, tonsillar, face or scalp infections)
2. Infectious mononucleosis (p. 72)
3. Tuberculosis or other mycobacterial infections
4. Secondary carcinoma (oral or nasopharyngeal primary)
5. (i) Hodgkin's disease
   (ii) Non-Hodgkin's lymphoma
   (iii) Leukaemia (esp. lymphocytic) (p. 110)

SALIVARY GLAND SWELLINGS (SUBMANDIBULAR OR LOWER
POLE OF PAROTID) (See p. 93)
1. Mumps
2. Tumours (particularly pleomorphic adenoma)
3. Sjögren's or sicca syndrome
4. Sarcoidosis
5. Suppurative parotitis

SWELLINGS OF SIDE OF NECK
1. Actinomycosis (p. 46)
2. Branchial cyst
3. Parapharyngeal cellulitis (p. 45)

MIDLINE SWELLING OF NECK
1. Thyroglossal cyst
2. Thyroid tumours or goitre
3. Deep ranula (p. 100)
4. Ludwig's angina (p. 45)

## HODGKIN'S DISEASE
1. Cervical lymph nodes most common first site (other lymphomas also frequently first affect cervical lymph nodes)
2. Any age affected, but most often young adult males
3. Nodes discrete — no invasion of surrounding tissues. Painless. Rubbery consistency
4. Patients initially well. Later fever, loss of weight, malaise, anaemia, pruritis. Infection (e.g. herpes zoster) due to depression of cell-mediated immunity occasionally first sign
5. Diagnosis by biopsy — essential for any persistently enlarged cervical nodes in absence of detectable cause
6. Pathology difficult. Mixed and variable cellular picture — lymphocytes, histiocytes and eosinophils. Reed-Sternberg giant cells characteristic. Classification based on histology
7. Treatment. Irradiation of localised disease. Chemotherapy for more advanced cases
8. 5-year survival rate over 80 per cent in patients with localised disease. Permanent cure possible in some
9. Hodgkin's disease of oral soft tissues exceedingly rare

## NON-HODGKIN'S LYMPHOMA ('LYMPHOSARCOMA')
1. Can cause enlarged cervical nodes, salivary gland swelling or (very rarely) an intraoral tumour. May be early manifestation or part of widespread disease
2. Typically nondescript soft swellings
3. Microscopically mostly of B lymphocyte origin
4. Usually tumour of mature, small B lymphocytes or follicle centre cells but many variants and classification controversial
5. Intracytoplasmic monoclonal immunoglobulin production may be detectable
6. Prognosis dependent on:
   (i) cell type
   (ii) extent of disease
7. 5-year survival rate about 30 per cent

# Pain and disorders of sensation or neuromuscular function

## PAIN

SUMMARY OF ORAL AND DENTAL CAUSES

### Teeth and supporting tissues
1. Pulpitis
2. Periapical periodontitis
3. Lateral (periodontal) abscess
4. Pericoronitis

### Oral mucosa
1. Herpes zoster
2. Carcinoma (later stages)
3. Tuberculosis
4. Mucosal ulceration (including ulcerative gingivitis) when exceptionally severe

### Jaws
1. Fractures
2. Osteomyelitis
3. Infected cysts
4. Malignant tumours

### The edentulous patient
1. Denture faults
2. Pressure on bony prominences
3. Disease of mucosa (as above) in denture-bearing area
4. Diseases of jaws (as above)
5. Teeth or roots erupting under denture

### Post-operative pain
1. Alveolar osteitis (dry socket)
2. Fracture of jaw
3. Osteomyelitis
4. Damage to nerve trunks ('traumatic neuroma')

**Pain on mastication**
1. Pain-dysfunction syndrome
2. TMJ disease
3. Temporal (giant cell) arteritis
4. Trigeminal neuralgia
5. Diseases of teeth and supporting tissues

SUMMARY OF PARA-ORAL AND EXTRA-ORAL CAUSES

**Disease of salivary glands**
1. Acute parotitis (bacterial and viral)
2. Severe Sjögren's syndrome
3. Malignant tumours

**Disease of the maxillary antrum**
1. Acute sinusitis
2. Cancer

**Pain of vascular origin**
1. Migrainous neuralgia
2. Temporal arteritis
3. Myocardial infarction

**Pain of neurological origin**
1. Trigeminal neuralgia
2. Herpes zoster
3. Post-herpetic neuralgia
4. Bell's palsy (in about 50 per cent of cases)
5. Multiple sclerosis
6. Intracranial tumours

**Psychogenic pain**
Atypical facial pain (usually associated with depression)

*Migrainous neuralgia*
1. Vasomotor instability of extracranial arteries, probably triggered by histamine
2. Pain typically deep to or around eye rarely in lower jaw
3. Vasomotor signs in face (reddening, oedema, watering eye, stuffy nose, etc.)
4. Sometimes regular onset at fixed time of day
5. Prolonged remissions common
6. Usually young adults: eventually self-limiting
7. Moderately good response to ergotamine

*Temporal arteritis*
1. Typically causes severe headache
2. Can cause severe ischaemic muscle pain on mastication or in tongue (p. 121)

*Myocardial infarction*
1. Pain can radiate to left arm and jaw — occasionally felt in left jaw only
2. Other effects of infarct usually apparent (p. 127)

*Trigeminal neuralgia*
1. Cause unknown; no objective signs
2. Typical features:
    (i) Affects trigeminal sensory area
    (ii) Pain paroxysmal, intense, lightning-like
    (iii) Trigger zones. Triggers include touch, cold or mastication
3. Elderly predominantly
4. Spontaneous temporary remissions common
5. Responds to anticonvulsants (carbamazepine)
6. Section of sensory root of trigeminal ganglion is treatment of last resort. Complications may be severe

*Bell's palsy*
Pain in jaw occasionally precedes palsy

*Herpes zoster of Vth nerve*
Toothache-like pain may be first symptom (p. 72)

*Post-herpetic neuralgia*
1. Mostly in elderly
2. Pain severe: persistent — not paroxysmal
3. Poor response to analgesics and anticonvulsants

*Multiple sclerosis*
1. Facial neuralgia uncommon; usually late
2. May mimic trigeminal neuralgia, or cause persistent pain

*Psychogenic (atypical) facial pain*
1. Features variable. Pain often felt in maxilla
2. Pain may be severe, persistent and unrelieved by analgesics
3. Physical cause for pain absent
4. Signs of depression may become apparent or be repressed
5. Delusional symptoms may be associated
6. May respond dramatically to antidepressant treatment
7. Occasionally complaint persists for years irrespective of treatment of any kind

## PARAESTHESIA AND ANAESTHESIA OF THE LIP
1. Inferior dental blocks
2. Trauma (fractures or operative damage)
3. Acute osteomyelitis
4. Malignant tumours of jaw
5. Pressure on mental nerve
6. Herpes zoster
7. Multiple sclerosis
8. Tetany

## FACIAL PALSY OR WEAKNESS
1. Bell's palsy
2. Stroke
3. Tumours (intracranial, parotid cancer, etc.)
4. Surgical damage
5. Head injury
6. Multiple sclerosis
7. Myasthenia gravis

# Systematic diseases affecting dentistry

1. Blood diseases
2. Cardiovascular disease
3. Endocrine disorders
4. Nutritional deficiencies
5. Hepatic, renal and miscellaneous

## BLOOD DISEASES

DEFECTS OF HAEMOSTASIS
1. Purpura (mainly platelet deficiencies or dysfunction)
2. Clotting defects

*Investigation*
*First* ask about
1. Duration of bleeding after previous extractions
2. Other haemorrhagic episodes
3. Management of previous haemorrhages (esp. if transfused)
4. Other operations (especially tonsillectomy)
5. Family history
6. Drugs (especially anticoagulants or aspirin)
7. Hospital card (e.g. for haemophilia)
Laboratory investigation of haemostasis if history suggests

PURPURA

*Causes*
1. Idiopathic thrombocytopenic (auto-immune)
2. Marrow diseases (especially acute leukaemia, aplastic anaemia)
3. Drugs (aspirin, chlorothiazide diuretics, apronal, etc.)
4. Scurvy
5. Vascular purpura (corticosteroids)

*Effects*
1. Spontaneous bruising (i.e. subcutaneous or submucosal bleeding)
2. Prolonged bleeding after extractions (usually stops spontaneously by clotting)
3. Severe gingival or nasal haemorrhages
4. Mucosal blood blisters

**Diagnosis**
1. Prolonged bleeding time
2. Tests of clotting function (see p. 109)
3. Manage according to underlying cause

CLOTTING DEFECTS
1. Deficiency of plasma factors usually VIII or IX
2. Hypoprothrombinaemia (impaired liver function, anticoagulants, vitamin K deficiency)
3. Hypofibrinogenaemia

**Haemophilia**
1. Sex-linked recessive (family history negative in about 30 per cent). About 1 in 10 000 males affected
   Haemophilia A (factor VIII deficiency) about 10 times commoner than haemophilia B (Christmas disease, IX deficiency)
2. Clinically and genetically, haemophilia A and B identical
3. Bleeding time normal but clotting grossly impaired
4. Delayed onset of persistent bleeding after injury (e.g. extraction)
5. Trauma (including local anaesthetic injections) causes *deep* soft tissue bleeding and haematomas
6. Haemarthroses in severe cases
7. Milder cases sometimes detected only as a result of dental treatment occasionally late in life

*Clinical aspects*
1. Management of extractions
   (i) Pre-operative radiographic dental assessment
   (ii) Admit to hospital
   (iii) Give adequate cryoprecipitate or AHF plus anti-fibrinolytic agent (tranexamic acid) or desmopressin (DDAVP)
   (iv) Keep under observation. Give more AHF if necessary
   (v) Give analgesic if necessary — *not* aspirin
   (vi) Make sure patient knows about risks of dental operations
2. Other complications
   (i) Haemorrhage from fractures
   (ii) Deep soft tissue bleeding due to local anaesthetic injections

## ANTICOAGULANT TREATMENT
1. Widely used for thromboembolic disease and disorders with risk of embolism, e.g. deep vein thrombosis, myocardial infarction, open heart surgery, etc.
2. With coumarin-type anticoagulants, dental surgery feasible if prothrombin time not more than 2 × control
3. Renal dialysis patients heparinised. Short acting; delay surgical treatment for 1 day after last dialysis

*Examples of important laboratory tests of clotting function*
1. Prothrombin Time — used in control of anticoagulant treatment
2. Partial Thromboplastin Time — detects deficiencies of factors VIII and IX and others
3. Thromboplastin Generation Test — distinguishes between factor VIII and IX deficiencies (but slow)
4. Factor VIII and IX assays — diagnostic and essential for management

*Note*: Whole blood clotting time — little or no practical value — normal in at least 25 per cent of haemophiliacs

## VON WILLEBRAND'S DISEASE
1. Autosomal dominant
2. Abnormal platelet function, prolonged bleeding time and factor VIII deficiency
3. Usually manifested as purpura rather than clotting defect
4. Prolonged bleeding from minor cuts or dental operations. Nosebleeds common
5. Bleeding greatly prolonged by aspirin. Dental bleeding often controllable by local pressure or suturing
6. Severe cases may need whole blood, platelet concentrates of cryoprecipitate

## ANAEMIA

*Causes*
1. Iron deficiency
2. Macrocytic (B$_{12}$ or folate deficiency)
3. Secondary
    (i) Leukaemia
    (ii) Malabsorption syndromes
    (iii) Drugs

*Dental implications*
1. Glossitis or angular cheilitis
2. Aphthous stomatitis occasionally
3. Infections (severe anaemia)
4. Hypoxia (and related complications) during anaesthesia

**Diagnosis**
1. Full blood picture
2. Investigate and (if possible) remedy cause of anaemia

## SICKLE CELL TRAIT AND ANAEMIA
1. Sickle cell trait (heterozygotes). Haemolysis precipitated by hypoxia
2. Sickle cell anaemia (homozygotes — rare). Admit to hospital for treatment

## POLYCYTHAEMIA VERA
1. Haemorrhagic tendencies
2. Cyanosis (without hypoxia)

## ACUTE LEUKAEMIA
1. Children — usually acute lymphocytic
   Adults — usually myelomonocytic
2. General effects
   (i) Anaemia
   (ii) Bleeding (thrombocytopenia)
   (iii) Infections
3. Oral features
   (i) Mucosal pallor
   (ii) Gingival bleeding, mucosal purpura
   (iii) Gingival swelling (adults)
   (iv) Gingival or mucosal ulceration (aggravated by cytotoxic drugs) — rigorous oral hygiene essential
4. Enlarged lymph nodes

## CHRONIC LEUKAEMIA
1. Typically insidious. Mild fever, weight loss, malaise and anorexia. Asymptomatic in 15 per cent
2. Oral lesions often absent
3. Occasionally oral purpura, infections and signs of anaemia

**Diagnosis**
1. Full blood picture
2. Marrow biopsy

## MYELOMA (See p. 59)

## APLASTIC ANAEMIA
1. Idiopathic (? auto-immune)
2. Drugs (chloramphenicol, phenylbutazone, etc.)
3. Irradiation

*Effects*
1. Anaemia
2. Infections
3. Bleeding

## AGRANULOCYTOSIS
1. Often drug-associated (phenylbutazone, phenothiazines, cotrimoxazole, antithyroid agents)
2. Effects — infections (especially gingival and pharyngeal ulceration)

## CYCLIC NEUTROPENIA
1. Diminution in neutrophils in 3 to 4 week cycles
2. Associated susceptibility to infection — mainly dermal or mucosal (gingival or pharyngeal) painful ulceration or
3. Rapid periodontal destruction
4. Rarely authenticated

## CARDIOVASCULAR DISEASE

### HYPERTENSION AND ISCHAEMIC HEART DISEASE

*Hazards*
1. Infarction or re-infarction during anaesthesia
2. Cardiac arrest (various precipitating factors)
3. Interaction of antihypertensive drugs with general anaesthetics
4. Dysrhythmias due to adrenaline in local anaesthetics if overdose given
5. Acute hypertension due to noradrenaline
6. Bleeding due to anticoagulant treatment

*Aspects of management*
1. Prevent pain and anxiety
2. Avoid general anaesthesia. Sedation may be feasible
3. Give adequate (not excessive) amounts of local anaesthetic
4. Aspirating syringe — theoretical advantages only
5. No clinically proven advantages of felypressin over adrenaline in local anaesthetic. *Do not use noradrenaline*

## ANGINA PECTORIS
1. Acute episodes of severe chest pain (myocardial ischaemia) typically precipitated by exercise or emotion
2. Pain usually relieved by rest and vasodilators (e.g. nitrates)
3. For angina during dental treatment, let patient use own vasodilator — if pain persists patient may have had an infarct (see below)

## HEART FAILURE

*Hazards*
1. Exacerbation or cardiac arrest under general anaesthesia
2. Problems related to cause of failure (e.g. hypertension, cardiac ischaemia or valve disease)

*Aspects of management*
1. Avoid general anaesthetic
2. Manage according to underlying cause (e.g. hypertension, valve disease, etc.)

## VALVE DISEASE

*Hazards*
1. Infective endocarditis
2. Problems due to effects of valve disease (e.g. failure)

*Aspects of management*
1. Antimicrobial prophylaxis for extractions or deep scaling
2. If in heart failure, manage accordingly

## INFECTIVE ENDOCARDITIS

*Cardiac lesions susceptible to infection*
1. Chronic rheumatic valve disease
2. Congenital defects
3. Prosthetic heart valves
4. Other disorders including calcific aortic degeneration

*Causes of bacteraemia*
1. Dental procedures but particularly extractions and deep scaling
2. Many other, non-dental, sources of infection, e.g. cardiac surgery, intravascular catheters, etc.

*Microbiology*
1. Mainly viridans streptococci, rarely enterococci, of dental origin
2. Severity of bacteraemia related to degree of gingival sepsis
3. Many other microbial causes (not from mouth)

*Dentistry as a precipitating cause of infective endocarditis*
1. Other, non-dental, risk factors (e.g. medical procedures, drug addiction, etc.) currently more important
2. Relevant dental history in only 6 to 10 per cent of cases
3. Peak incidence now *after age 60* due to non-dental risk factors

*Mortality*
1. 5 to 15 per cent for viridans streptococcal infections, if adequately treated
2. Overall mortality about 30 per cent, due to virulent, non-dental, infections (e.g. staphylococcal, fungal, etc.) and impaired host defences
3. High mortality in prosthetic valve endocarditis but infection rarely of dental origin

*Prevention*
1. Amoxycillin 3 g orally immediately pre-operatively for patients at risk (if not allergic to penicillin) or oral erythromycin
2. No prophylactic regime *known* to be effective due to impossibility of conducting controlled trials
3. High-risk patients (especially if previous attacks of infective endocarditis) or if requiring general anaesthesia — refer to hospital for parenteral prophylaxis

## ENDOCRINE DISORDERS

PITUITARY

**Acromegaly**
1. Prognathism, increasing obliquity of angle, spacing of teeth, disordered occlusion
2. Macroglossia
3. Thickening of facial features
4. Spade-like extremities
5. Complications. Diabetes (70 per cent), hypertension (30 per cent), muscular weakness. Effects of cerebral tumour, especially on optic tracts
6. Treatment. Excision or irradiation of pituitary tumour

THYROID

**Thyrotoxicosis**
1. Irritability and nervousness
2. Tachycardia, dysrhythmias and heart failure
3. Risks of dysrhythmias with adrenaline in local anaesthetics (theoretically)

**Cretinism**
1. Dwarfism
2. Imbecility
3. Delayed eruption

**Myxoedema**
Ischaemic heart disease
See above, page 111)

## PARATHYROIDS

**Hyperparathyroidism**
Osteitis fibrosa cystica (p. 63)

**Hypoparathyroidism (idiopathic)**
1. Enamel hypoplasia (p. 65)
2. Chronic mucocutaneous candidosis (p. 81) occasionally

## ADRENALS

**Hypofunction (Addison's disease)**
1. Oral pigmentation
2. Collapse under general anaesthesia or other stress
3. Chronic mucocutaneous candidosis occasionally

**Complications of corticosteroid treatment**
1. Circulatory collapse under stress esp. general anaesthesia (p. 129)
2. Infections (e.g. oral candidosis)
3. Impaired healing
4. Osteoporosis
5. Life-threatening disease may be masked

## DIABETES MELLITUS
1. Infections (including periodontal)
2. Dry mouth if diabetes uncontrolled
3. Hypoglycaemic coma
4. Ketotic coma
5. Dangers during general anaesthesia

## NUTRITIONAL DISORDERS

*Note*: Nutritional deficiencies all now rare in Britain, but occasionally secondary to malabsorption. Only vitamin $B_{12}$, folate and iron deficiency (p. 109) seen in significant numbers

*Vitamin A deficiency*
1. Experimentally causes squamous change and keratosis of glandular epithelia
2. Main effect in man — night blindness and xerophthalmia
3. No proven contribution to oral leukoplakia
4. Reports of low vitamin A intake in head and neck cancer patients, but cancer-preventing effect of vitamin A largely speculative

*Vitamin B group*

*Thiamine deficiency*
Main effects — neuritis and cardiac failure

*Riboflavin deficiency*
1. Angular and generalised stomatitis
2. Tongue typically purplish and pebbly
3. Dermatitis

*Nicotinic acid deficiency — pellagra*
1. Glossitis sometimes with ulceration
2. Red, swollen gingivae
3. Sometimes generalised stomatitis
4. Weakness, loss of appetite, psychiatric disorders, gastrointestinal disturbance, dermatitis

*Vitamin $B_{12}$ deficiency*
Macrocytic anaemia and subacute combined degeneration of the cord (p. 109)

*Folate deficiency*
Macrocytic anaemia (p. 109)

*Vitamin C deficiency. Scurvy*
1. Virtually only of historical interest
2. Defective collagen formation
3. Purpura (platelet defect and weakened vessel walls), dermatitis, mental changes
4. In severe cases swollen, bleeding gums due to haemorrhagic tendency and defective collagen

*Vitamin D deficiency*
1. Mainly seen in Indian or Pakistani immigrants living in Northern cities as a result of marginal vitamin D and calcium intake, lack of exposure to sunshine and use of wholemeal flour (impairs calcium absorption) at times of high demand (pregnancy and growth)
2. Defective calcification especially at epiphyses leading to irregular proliferation of cartilage, connective tissue and blood vessels
3. Weakening and distortion of bones
4. Hypocalcification of dentine only in exceptionally severe cases

*Vitamin K deficiency*
1. Not nutritional
2. Caused by failure of synthesis by intestinal flora (haemorrhatic disease of the newborn) or interference with absorption (obstructive jaundice) or metabolism (anticoagulants or liver disease)
3. Clotting defect and bleeding tendency due to failure (mainly) of prothrombin formation

## HEPATIC, RENAL AND MISCELLANEOUS DISEASES

HEPATITIS B
1. Mainly transmitted parenterally especially by blood or blood products but also sexually or (occasionally) by saliva
2. High risks
   a. Renal dialysis
   b. Organ transplants
   c. Long-term immunosuppressive treatment
   d. Repeated tranfusions or injections of blood products (e.g. haemophiliacs)
   e. Institutions for the mentally handicapped (especially with Down's syndrome)
   f. Drug addiction
   g. History suggestive of hepatitis
   h. Patients from high-risk areas (e.g. many parts of Asia) especially after transfusions, tattooing, ear-piercing, etc. there
   i. Male homosexuals
   j. VD clinic patients
3. Immunological diagnosis
   (i) $HB_sAg$ present in active disease. Usually disappears with development of antibody about 4 months after onset
   (ii) Carriers. $HB_sAg$ persists
   (iii) $HB_cAg$ — present in virus core and nuclei of affected liver cells in early stages of disease
   (iv) The e antigen — associated with active disease
4. Inactivation of virus
   (i) Destroyed by autoclaving for 15 minutes at 121°C
   (ii) Dry heat, formaldehyde (40 per cent) or hypochlorite (10 per cent) also effective but slower
5. Management
   (i) Have suspected carriers tested for antigen
   (ii) When treating carriers
      a. Wear gloves, eyeshield and mask
      b. Autoclave all instuments or use disposables
      c. Do not re-use LA cartridges (as in any patient)
      d. Use low-speed instruments
6. Treatment. HB immune globulin may give protection after exposure. Active immunisation with $HB_sAg$ vaccine for high risk of exposure

## CROHN'S DISEASE
1. Chronic inflammation with 'tuberculoid' granulomas. Typically, cobblestone proliferation of mucosa especially of ileocaecal region, ulceration, fibrosis, malabsorption, fistulas, pain
2. Pebbly or cobblestone proliferation of oral mucosa with same histopathology as gut. May precede gut lesions
3. Malabsorption, especially $B_{12}$ or folate deficiency, may also affect mouth
4. Increased frequency of aphthous stomatitis (unconfirmed) may be associated with folate deficiency or ragged oral ulcers

## SARCOIDOSIS
1. Multiple, noncaseating 'tuberculoid' granulomas especially of lung
2. Cause unknown. Partial anergy (defect of cell-mediated immunity), e.g. tuberculin negative
3. Oral lesions
    (i) Salivary gland swelling (about 5 per cent)
    (ii) Heerfordt's syndrome. Fever, parotid swelling, uveitis, facial and other cranial nerve palsies
    (iii) Gingival swelling

**Diagnosis**
1. Biopsy
2. Chest radiographs
3. Kveim test

## RENAL DISEASE
1. Dialysis patients. Risks of hepatitis B and bleeding due to heparinisation
2. Transplant patients. Complications of immunosuppressive treatment. Usually also risks associated with preceding dialysis (e.g. hepatitis B)
3. Renal failure (untreated). Stomatitis. Susceptibility to infection. Bleeding. 'Uraemic halitosis'
4. Impaired renal function. Tetracyclines may precipitate failure. Vancomycin, aminoglycosides, amphotericin, phenacetin (and other drugs) also nephrotoxic
5. Renal failure sometimes associated with leukoplakia-like oral white lesions which resolve with effective dialysis or transplant

# Immunological aspects of oral disease and immunologically-mediated diseases of dental relevance

*Review of basic immunology*
Basic immune responses to antigens
1. Humoral (antibody production)
   Dependent on plasma cells, the progeny of B lymphocytes.
   Protective antibodies are IgM, IgG or IgA (in secretions)
2. Cell-mediated
   Dependent on T lymphocytes (producing lymphokines) and macrophages

*Consequences of immune responses*
1. Protection against infections — their main 'purpose'
2. Can activate complement-enhancing inflammatory response — usually also protective
3. Can mediate hypersensitivity reactions leading to immunologically-mediated disease, i.e. defective *control* of otherwise normal immune responses (see below)

*Abnormal immune function*
1. Inadequate immune response
   Immunodeficiency states
2. Abnormal immune reactions
   a. Response to *foreign* antigens may be excessive or provoke IgE production
   b. As a result of loss of self-tolerance may respond to *host* tissues as antigens (auto-immune reactions)

**Hypersensivity reactions**

*Type 1 immediate*
   (i) IgE production in response to antigen (allergen)
   (ii) IgE + allergen cause release of mediators from mast cells.
       Clinical manifestations: Atopic allergy and anaphylaxis (see
       below)

*Type 2 cytotoxic*
T lymphocytes (with antibodies or complement) directly cytotoxic
   Clinical example: Thrombocytopenic purpura (anti-platelet
antibodies)

*Type 3 Immune complex reactions*
Persistence of immune complexes (Ag/Ab), activation of
complement, chemotaxis of neutrophils and tissue damage by
neutrophil enzymes
   Clinical examples: Serum sickness, vasculitis. (Immune complex
mechanism rarely however confirmable with certainty)

*Type 4 cell-mediated reactions*
T lymphocytes (activated by antigen) produce lymphokines which
attract macrophages and other effector cells to attack antigen
   (Cell-mediated 'Immunity' and cell-mediated 'Hypersensitivity'
depend on the same mechanisms and not distinguishable in
practical terms)
   Clinical examples: Tuberculin reaction, contact dermatitis, some
transplant rejection mechanisms

   *Note:* Though Type 4 reactions are termed 'hypersensitivity' (i.e.
harmful) reactions, *absence* of such reactions (anergy) is associated
with abnormal susceptibility to infection

IMMUNOLOGICALLY-MEDIATED DISEASES
1. Reactions to *exogenous* antigens
   Atopic allergy and anaphylaxis (type 1 reaction)
   Contact dermatitis (type 4 reaction)
   Transplant rejection (type 4 and other reactions)
2. Reactions to *host* antigens (loss of self-tolerance)
   Auto-immune diseases
   a. *Mediated by organ or cell specific auto-antibodies* Idiopathic
      thrombocytopenic purpura, Hashimoto's thyroiditis,
      pemphigus vulgaris, Addison's disease
   b. *Lacking organ-specific auto-antibodies* (thought to be immune
      complex-mediated) The connective tissue diseases; Sjögren's
      syndrome, rheumatoid arthritis, systemic lupus erythematosus

## TYPICAL FEATURES OF AUTO-IMMUNE DISEASE
1. Women more commonly affected
2. Family history often positive
3. Hypergammaglobulinaemia due to circulating auto-antibodies often detectable
4. Multiple auto-antibodies produced but many without clinical effects
5. Circulating auto-antibodies may be detectable in relatives also without clinical effects
6. Tissues under attack infiltrated by lymphocytes in some (e.g. Sjögren's syndrome)
7. Vasculitis and arthritis typical of immune complex disorders (e.g. rheumatoid arthritis and systemic lupus erythematosus)
8. Immunoglobulin and complement may be detectable at site of tissue damage in some (e.g. pemphigus vulgaris) by immunofluorescence microscopy
9. Responds to immunosuppressive treatment (if organ damage is not complete)

## IMMEDIATE TYPE HYPERSENSITIVITY AND ATOPIC ALLERGY
1. IgE mediated. Strong familial susceptibility
2. About 10 per cent of population affected
3. Manifestations — asthma, eczema, urticaria, hay-fever, food allergies, drug reactions
4. Minor effects, only, controlled by antihistamines
5. Dental aspects
   (i) Drug allergy and anaphylaxis
   (ii) Anaesthetic and other hazards of asthma
   (iii) Acute urticaria — risk of oedema of glottis
   (iv) Risks of corticosteroid treatment (e.g. for severe asthma)
   (v) Antihistamines — dry mouth, potentiate sedating agents
6. No evidence of oral disease due to immediate-type hypersensitivity

## CONNECTIVE TISSUE (COLLAGEN VASCULAR) DISEASES

### Rheumatoid arthritis
1. 1 to 3 per cent of population affected, women particularly
2. Inflammation, pain and swelling of small joints especially, symmetrically. With variable other multisystem effects
3. Can affect TMJ. Effects usually minor
4. Sjögren's syndrome in about 15 per cent
5. Possible oral reactions to drugs used for treatment, e.g. aspirin, gold corticosteroids
6. Immunological features:
   (i) Increased Rheumatoid Factor (anti-IgG) in serum in 75 per cent
   (ii) LE cell positive in 10 to 30 per cent
   (iii) Immune complexes and complement activation especially in joints

**Sjögren's syndrome**
See Page 96

**Systemic lupus erythematosus (SLE)**
1. Mucocutaneous lesions. Occasionally first sign
2. Oral lesions — white patches and erosions in about 20 per cent. Generally resistant to topical treatment
3. Histopathology of mucosal lesions
    (i) Variable acanthosis, thinning or ulceration of epithelium
    (ii) Liquefaction degeneration of basal cell layer
    (iii) Thickening of basement membrane (PAS positive)
    (iv) Variable, scattered, mainly lymphocytic, infiltrate in connective tissue
    (v) Vasculitis *may* be seen in systemic (not discoid) LE
4. Butterfly rash on face
5. May be on corticosteroid treatment
6. Sjögren's syndrome in 30 per cent (estimated)
7. Multisystem disease (arthralgia, renal, neuro-psychiatric, cardiac or pulmonary lesions)
8. Thrombocytopenia (with bleeding) in some
9. Immunological features and aspects of diagnosis
    (i) Anti-nuclear antibodies (95+ per cent but titres unrelated to clinical severity)
    (ii) Positive LE cell phenomenon (75 to 80 per cent)
    (iii) Rheumatoid factor in nearly 30 per cent
    (iv) Hypocomplementaemia
    (v) Anti-RBC and /or platelets (70 to 80 per cent)
    (vi) Immunoglobulin and complement deposited along basement membrane beneath lesions and normal epithelium

**Discoid lupus erythematosus**
1. Predominantly mucocutaneous
2. Oral lesions and cutaneous lesions essentially similar to SLE. May mimic lichen planus
3. Diagnosis — biopsy (see SLE above)
4. Immunological features
    (i) Immunoglobulin and complement deposited along basement membrane under lesions only
    (ii) No significant serological changes

**Cranial (giant cell) arteritis**
1. Relatively common in elderly
2. Obliterative arteritis with giant cells in media, especially small arteries at base of skull
3. Occasionally severe ischaemic muscle pain during mastication. Rarely, ischaemic necrosis of tongue
4. Typically sudden headache with prominent tender, tortuous temporal arteries
5. Risk of optic atrophy. Good response to corticosteroids. Must be given because of danger to sight

**Diagnosis**
1. High ESR
2. Temporal artery biopsy

**Wegener's granulomatosis**
1. Necrotising arteritis. Widespread chronic inflammation with giant cells in affected sites
2. Granulomatous gingivitis occasionally first sign
3. Renal damage may be fatal

**Diagnosis**
1. Biopsy
2. Renal function tests

**Progressive systemic sclerosis (scleroderma)**
1. Overproduction of subepithelial collagen
2. Leathery stiffening of skin and viscera, especially oesophagus (dysphagia). Mask-like immobile facies
3. Widening of periodontal membrane shadow (about 7 per cent)
4. Sjögren's syndrome in 5 per cent
5. Opening of mouth may be limited, but oral effects often minor
6. Renal damage typically fatal
7. Immunological features:
    (i) Hypergammaglobulinaemia frequently
   (ii) Rheumatoid factor in 25 to 30 per cent
   (iii) Anti-nuclear antibodies in 70 per cent

IMMUNOLOGICALLY-MEDIATED DISEASES RELEVANT TO
DENTISTRY — SUMMARY
1. Reactions to exogenous antigens
   Atopic allergy and anaphylaxis (type 1 reactions)
   (Contact dermatitis (type 4 reactions) — mucosa probably not
   affected)
2. 'Auto-immune' disease
   The connective tissue diseases
     Rheumatoid arthritis
     Sjögren's and sicca syndromes* (p. 96)
     Lupus erythematosus*
     Systemic sclerosis*
     Wegener's granulomatosis*
     Giant cell (temporal) arteritis
   Mucocutaneous diseases
     Pemphigus vulgaris* (p. 77)
     Mucous membrane pemphigoid* (p. 77)
   Gastrointestinal disease
     Chronic atrophic gastritis and pernicious anaemia
     Coeliac disease
   Haematological disease
     Pernicious anaemia* (p. 109)
     Idiopathic and drug-associated thrombocytopenic purpura*
     (p. 107)
     Drug-associated leucopenia
     Auto-immune haemolytic anaemia
   Endocrine disease
     Addison's disease* (p. 114)
     Hypothyroidism (Hashimoto's thyroiditis)
     Hyperthyroidism
     Idiopathic hypoparathyroidism* (p. 114)

*Have characteristic oral manifestations

## IMMUNODEFICIENCIES

The chief effect of immune-deficiency is increased susceptibility to infection

1. Most common types
   (i) IgA deficiency
   (ii) Immunosuppressive treatment
   (iii) Down's syndrome
2. Severe genetic or developmental B and/or T cell disorders rare
3. IgA deficiency
   (i) Many healthy. Deficiency found fortuitously *or*
   (ii) Severe atopic allergy or
   (iii) Susceptibility to infection, especially respiratory or
   (iv) Connective tissue disease
   (v) Susceptibility to caries and periodontal disease — conflicting findings, *no* major effect on mouth
4. Immunosuppressive treatment
   (i) Cell-mediated immunity mainly affected
   (ii) Highly susceptible to infection (often opportunistic) — main cause of death
   (iii) Oral herpes and thrush common and severe but rarely disseminate
   (iv) Signs of inflammation (e.g. gingivitis) typically suppressed by anti-inflammatory action of drugs
   (v) Hepatitis B more common
   (vi) Circulatory collapse under stress (e.g. general anaesthesia) if unprotected by corticosteroid supplementation
5. Down's syndrome (Mongolism)
   (i) Defects of both cell-mediated and humoral immunity
   (ii) Mental defect, congenital anomalies (especially heart). Occlusal defects and hypodontia
   (iii) Susceptibility to infection (usual cause of early death in the past)
   (iv) High risk of hepatitis B if institutionalised
   (v) Typically, gross plaque accumulation, rapidly destructive periodontal disease but low caries activity
6. Severe defects of T cells and combined defects (e.g. Swiss-type agammaglobulinaemia, Di George syndrome)
   (i) Greatly increased susceptibility to many infections
   (ii) Chronic oral candidosis common
   (iii) Often early death from infections

## ACQUIRED IMMUNE DEFICIENCY SYNDROME (AIDS)
1. First reported 1981
2. Several thousand cases in US, especially New York and San Francisco. Thought to be doubling in incidence every 6 months
3. Some cases from Haiti and Africa. A few in Europe
4. Promiscuous male homosexuals and intravenous drug addicts mainly affected
5. Others at risk — recipients of blood products (haemophiliacs), immigrants from Haiti and some parts of Africa, consorts of any of these
6. Cause unknown but thought to be a transmissible agent, probably a virus. Incubation period may be several years
7. Severe defect of cell-mediated immunity. Irreversible depression of T helper to T suppressor cell ratio. Humoral responses less affected
8. Wide range of opportunistic infections — bacterial, fungal, viral and protozoal otherwise only seen in deeply immunosuppressed patients
9. High frequency of unusual neoplasms particularly Kaposi's sarcoma (a malignant tumour of blood vessels) and lymphomas — also seen in deeply immunosuppressed patients (p. 91)
10. High frequency of oral lesions, especially Kaposi's sarcoma, carcinoma, chronic candidosis keratoses
11. No effective treatment known
12. Mortality: probably 80 per cent die within 3 years of diagnosis

## IMMUNOLOGICAL ASPECTS OF DENTAL DISEASE

*Dental caries*
1. Poor access of antigens to immunogenic tissues
2. Secretory IgA the only immune product reaching the teeth in significant amounts
3. Traces only of IgG and IgM reach mouth from gingival inflammatory exudate
4. Existence of natural immunity to caries controversial
5. Effect of immunodeficiency on caries activity — inconsistent findings but low caries incidence in Down's syndrome with multiple immunodeficiencies. (See also p. 15)

*Periodontal disease*
1. Gingival inflammation probably mediated by complement activation by endotoxins and antigen/antibody complexes
2. Strong antibody response to plaque indicated by local concentration of plasma cells and immunoglobulins in gingival tissues
3. No microscopic features suggestive of cytotoxic, immune complex or cell-mediated damage to supporting tissues
4. Immune response largely, therefore, protective and greatly retards tissue destruction in presence of massive infection
5. Immunodeficiency states (e.g. uncontrolled diabetes mellitus and Down's syndrome) lead to greatly accelerated periodontal destruction (See also p. 28)

*Periapical periodontitis*
1. Immune response (antibody production) detectable locally
2. Immune response appears to help to localise infection (the usual consequence of infection reaching this area)
3. No microscopic features suggestive of immunologically-mediated tissue damage (See also p. 21)

# APPENDIX
# Medical emergencies in dentistry

1. Fainting
2. Myocardial infarction
3. Cardiac arrest
4. Anaesthetic accidents
5. Acute anaphylactic reactions
6. Circulatory failure in patients on long-term corticosteroids
7. Other drug reactions and interactions
8. Epilepsy and status epilepticus
9. Status asthmaticus
10. Acute hypoglycaemia
11. Haemorrhage
12. Severe maxillo-facial injuries
13. Hysterical reactions

## FAINTING

1. Transient fall in blood pressure and cerebral ischaemia
2. Usually premonitory dizziness, confusion, nausea or vomiting
3. Pallor, cold damp skin
4. Depth of unconsciousness variable — rarely, incontinence or minor convulsion
5. Pulse initially slow then full and rapid
6. Lower head
7. Prevention — diazepam orally or i.v. sedation for regular fainters

## MYOCARDIAL INFARCTION

1. Mainly males. Typically middle-aged or over
2. May be hypertensive or past history of chest pain
3. May be precipitated by pain or anxiety
4. Agonisingly severe and persistent chest pain, often breathlessness; sometimes vomiting and shock
5. Make sure patient can breathe freely. Do *not* lie flat if breathing difficult due to pulmonary oedema
6. Give oxygen
7. Give morphine (10 to 20 mg) *not* pentazocine by injection *or*

127

8. Give $N_2O : O_2$ 50 : 50. Make sure airway is protected
9. Give constant reassurance
10. Call ambulance

## CARDIAC ARREST

1. Main causes
   (i) Myocardial infarction
   (ii) Hypoxia (e.g. during anaesthesia)
   (iii) Anaesthesia (but mainly with halogenated hydrocarbons during major abdominal or chest surgery)
   (iv) Severe hypotension (anaphylaxis or any other cause of circulatory collapse)
2. Be alert to risk of arrest especially in above circumstances particularly in patients with heart disease. Take precautions accordingly
3. Signs of arrest:
   (i) Loss of consciousness
   (ii) Absence of pulses
   (DO NOT wait for dilatation of pupils, lack of blood pressure, etc.)
4. Treat immediately
   (i) Lay patient supine
   (ii) Give 1 or 2 *sharp* blows with side of fist on midsternum (*may* restart heart or stop ventricular fibrillation)*
   (iii) Get help
   (iv) Clear the airway and keep clear. Hold jaw forward with neck extended
   (v) Start external cardiac compression immediately
   (vi) Give artificial ventilation intermittently (mouth to mouth)
   (vii) Get assistant to call ambulance (as soon as emergency measures started)
   (viii) Recovery: spontaneous pulse, improved colour, return of reflexes (e.g. contraction of pupils and blinking), spontaneous purposive movements
   (ix) Persist until specialist help available or for at least 15 minutes

## ANAESTHETIC ACCIDENTS

1. Respiratory obstruction
2. Failure of $O_2$ supply
3. Overdose of anaesthetic agent (especially intravenous barbiturates)
4. Respiratory failure (usually secondary to 1 to 3 above)
5. Cardiac arrest
6. Anaphylactic reactions to intravenous anaesthetics
7. Circulatory failure in patients on long-term corticosteroids or secondary to any of the above

* NOTE. Value controversial as precordial thump may also precipitate fibrillation

## ACUTE ANAPHYLAXIS

1. Main causes in dentistry
   (i) Penicillin
   (ii) Intravenous anaesthetic agents
2. Typical signs: paraesthesia of face, oedema, wheezing, flushing of skin, sudden loss of consciousness, (or deepening of unconsciousness) weak or impalpable pulse, low or unmeasurable blood pressure
3. Give intramuscular adrenaline (1ml of 1: 1000) then hydrocortisone succinate, 100 to 300 mg i.v. immediately
4. Lay patient flat. *Raise legs*
5. Call ambulance
6. Make sure patient has card indicating sensitivity to drug

## CIRCULATORY COLLAPSE IN PATIENTS ON LONG-TERM CORTICOSTEROIDS

1. Susceptible patients — any on long-term corticosteroids (and possibly for up to 2 years thereafter) irrespective of dose
2. Precipitating events:
   (i) General anaesthesia
   (ii) Surgery (multiple extractions or more major operations)
   (iii) Trauma
3. Loss of consciousness (or deepening unconsciousness) ashen pallor, loss of pulses, damp cold skin
4. Give hydrocortisone succinate 500 mg i.v.
5. Lay patient flat. *Raise legs*
6. Call ambulance
7. Repeat i.v. hydrocortisone if necessary after 10 minutes

## OTHER IMPORTANT DRUG REACTIONS OR INTERACTIONS

1. Noradrenaline (in local anaesthetic) — acute hypertension causing acute severe headache, stroke or death
2. Intravenous anaesthetic agents — overdose or hypersensitivity
3. Monoamine oxidase inhibitors — interaction with narcotic analgesics especially *pethidine*

## EPILEPSY

1. Rapid sequence of:
   (i) Sudden loss of consciousness
   (ii) Generalised muscular contraction (tonic phase)
   (iii) Generalised jerking movements (clonic phase)
   (iv) Recovery but prolonged drowsiness
2. Try to prevent tongue being bitten
3. Protect patient from injury on surrounding objects
4. Otherwise no treatment for attack itself
5. Make sure patient is escorted home or send to hospital

STATUS EPILEPTICUS
1. Repeated attacks in quick succession — can be fatal
2. Give diazepam i.v. (20 mg)
3. Call ambulance

## STATUS ASTHMATICUS

1. Persistent severe bronchospasm (wheezing and dyspnoea)
2. Give 300 mg hydrocortisone succinate *and* (if possible)
3. Aminophylline up to 375 mg i.v. *over 20 minutes, or*
4. Salbutamol 4g/kg very slowly i.v.
5. Give $O_2$
6. Call ambulance

## ACUTE HYPOGLYCAEMIA

1. Diabetics on insulin (overdose or missing a meal)
2. Clinically resembles fainting
3. Give sugar (six lumps in a drink) in premonitory stage
4. Lay patient flat (but does not cause recovery)
5. When unconscious, i.v. (sterile) glucose or intramuscular
   adrenaline (1 ml of 1:1000) effective

## HAEMORRHAGE (DENTAL)

1. Rarely dangerous (unless due to haemophilia)
2. Clear clot from mouth and find source of bleeding
3. Give local anaesthetic and suture
4. Get history especially of any other episodes or family history
5. If patient has haemophilia (or other haemorrhagic disease)
   (i) Control bleeding as well as possible with pressure pad and
       barrel bandage
   (ii) Admit immediately to hospital for antihaemophilic globulin (or
        other appropriate treatment)

## SEVERE MAXILLO-FACIAL INJURIES

1. *Make sure of airway* (remove foreign bodies, etc.)
2. Maintain airway
   (i) Pull tongue forward
   (ii) Lay patient on side
   (iii) Keep chin extended
3. Admit to hospital with airway under control

## HYSTERICAL REACTIONS

1. Reactions bizarre or inappropriate, typically exaggerated and theatrical
2. Manner may be obviously neurotic before start of treatment
3. Reactions to (e.g) local anaesthetic often reproduced by injection of normal saline
4. Sometimes paraesthesia or loss of sensation in non-anatomical distribution
5. Overbreathing may induce tetany and convulsions (p. 69)

# Index

133